SGT. OTTO

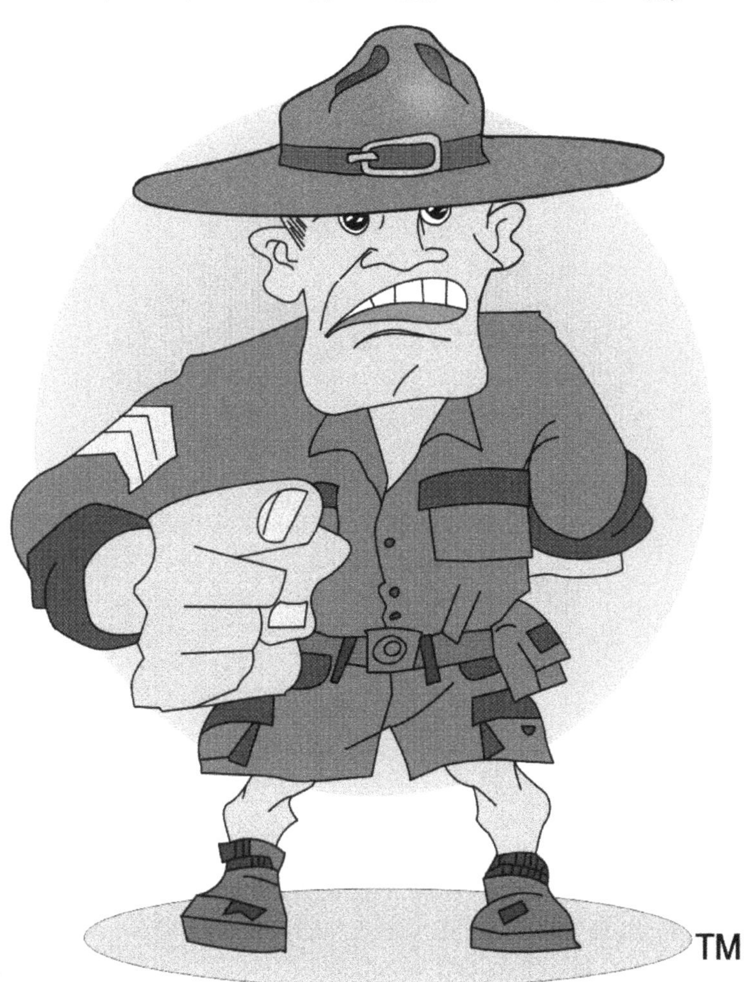

Man Diet

Sergeant Otto Man Diet

Weight Loss

Guaranteed

Fun

Written and Illustrated by

Lonnie Otto

Published by:

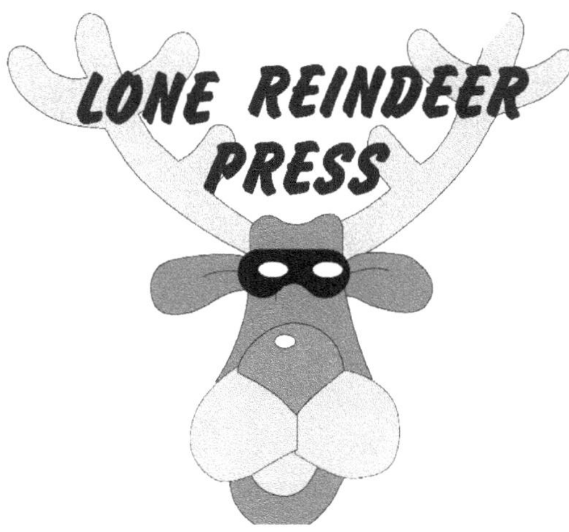

The reader should consult with a physician before embarking on any diet change that may affect existing or create new health conditions. Neither the author nor the publisher is liable to any reader for damages either direct or indirect arising from use of the information contained within. This book is written as a work of humor and entertainment. The reader takes sole responsibility for adopting or incorporating any of the suggestions contained within.

Every attempt has been made to identify owners of copyrighted material. Any errors or omissions will be immediately addressed and acknowledgments listed at www.sgtotto.com. Brand names, products cited, trademarks, and copyrights remain property of their owners.

Second printing, April 2015

Illustrated by Lonnie Otto

Published by: Lone Reindeer Press

Library of Congress Control Number: 2013946435

Otto, Lonnie
Sergeant Otto Man Diet

ISBN: 978-0-9897619-3-2
1. Health & Fitness-Weight Loss

Contact at www.sgtotto.com

Acknowledgments—PLEASE Read!

If all the advisors that contributed to Sergeant Otto Man Diet were listed in my "thank you," this section would exceed the length of the entire book! So if your name isn't listed below, well, tough shit! Besides, no one wants to read a long list of names of people they don't know.

However, there are a few major supporters who are now forever connected to this literary masterpiece. Without these individuals and their extensive military history and experiences, Sergeant Otto Man Diet would never have happened. They are:

C. L. M. Slagel, Commander, United States Navy, Retired
J. Slagel, Senior Special Agent NCIS, Retired/former Gunnery Sergeant, USMC
J. Slagel, Chemical, Biological, Nuclear Specialist, Lance Corporal, USMC Reserve

Sorry to have interrupted your family dinners for the umpteenth time. You can now eat in peace. Through our fifteen years of raising our kids, Katrina, leather jacket, barn doors, Israel, Gumby, Kayci, Elia and Sergeant Otto, I have come to understand the true meaning of "blood brothers."

And that Lucy—what a cutesy! You put the frosting on my cake!

To my kids—if twenty- and thirty-year-olds can still be called kids. For my son Jamie, your adult athleticism provided the inspiration—I did not want to be a fatso anymore. For my daughters Amber and Harlee, listen to your dad one more time. DO NOT READ FURTHER! After my next book, you will be proud to say, "That's my dad." Unfortunately, with this current publication I may have embarrassed you one more time. Sorry, girls. Are you mad?

And last to my beautiful wife of twenty-five years, affectionately known as Oooch, for enduring me as a fat slob for many years and now helping me recover from one of the most serious ailments known to mankind—lack-a-nookie. On Sunday mornings in bed when I hear from you "oh my God, OH MY GOD" I hope the good Lord will equate this with the same as attending church! Thank you, Jesus! And thank you, Oooch! Now that I am a skinny dude, you make me feel twenty-five years young! Without your tolerance and suggestions, this soon-to-be classic would never have seen the light of day!

Very fun for all...!

DEDICATION—MUST READ!

Now brief serious stuff—dedication to Mr. John (Sully) Sullivan.

Since graduation from the University of Connecticut over twenty years ago, John has worked tirelessly at local and federal agencies (currently through the Veterans Administration) to assist homeless veterans in overcoming personal difficulties and struggles.

Mr. Sullivan has been instrumental in providing housing, jobs, food, and medical assistance for THOUSANDS of veterans! For Mr. Sullivan this is not a 9-5 job but a 24/7 "calling." This dedication is a minimal footnote compared to his passionate commitment.

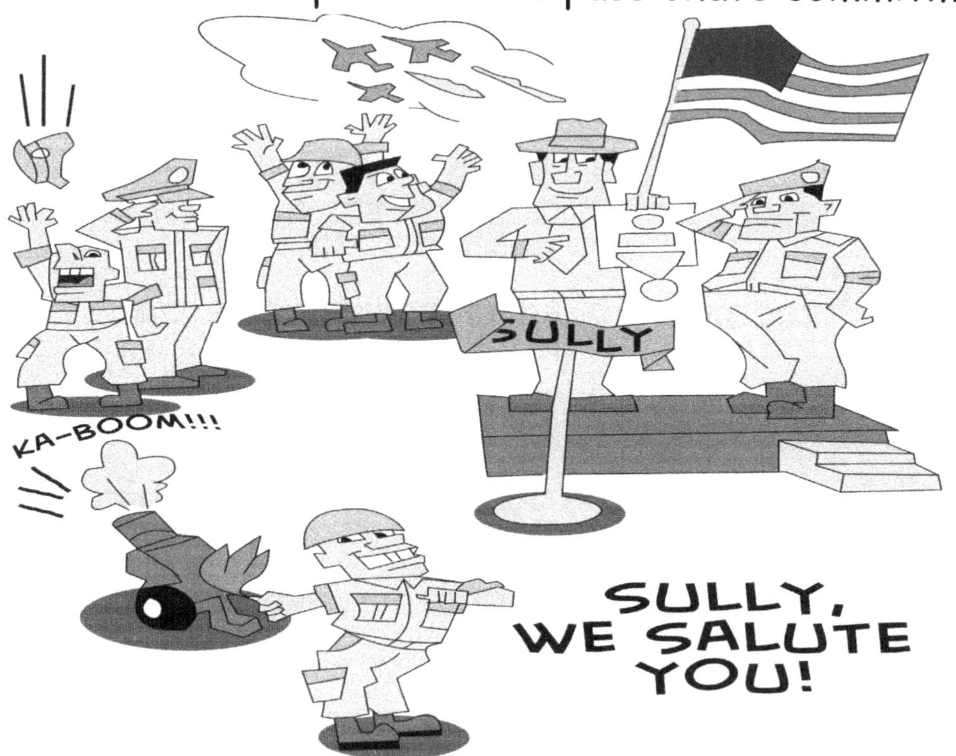

During the same twenty years conversing with John about his clients, my daily, sedentary routine resulted in a minuscule average weight gain of one-third of a pound per month. No biggie, right? Well, yes, biggie—about 80 pounds of biggie! Do the math. Two hundred and forty months, a third of a pound per month, **80 pounds**. I knew I was no supermodel, but I also never equated my weight to that of an NFL lineman!

After years of John "counseling" me about being a phatso, well CLICK, the light switch finally came on.

"Slow learner better than no learner," John often said to me.

John's jokes and jabs about my weight were the stimulus for me to assess my eating habits. Finally tired of his comments (spelled b-i-t-c-h-i-n-g), in less than eight months, I lost 80 pounds. I removed the equivalent of a bag of concrete strapped to my back, which I had carried around every day and night, year after year.

NOW IT IS TIME FOR YOU, CHUBBY,
TO GET THAT FAT BUTT IN GEAR!

We live in the "land-o-plenty." Our country has more food than any other and has more written about ways to eat it **AND** ways to keep from eating it.

I hope you'll find this weight loss guide entertaining as well as informative. Maybe this book can do for you what John did for me—turn your light switch on—to a healthier and sexier lifestyle.

If you weigh a ton,
You and Sgt. Otto have a lot to get done!

CONTENTS

Chapter 1
Got Gonads?

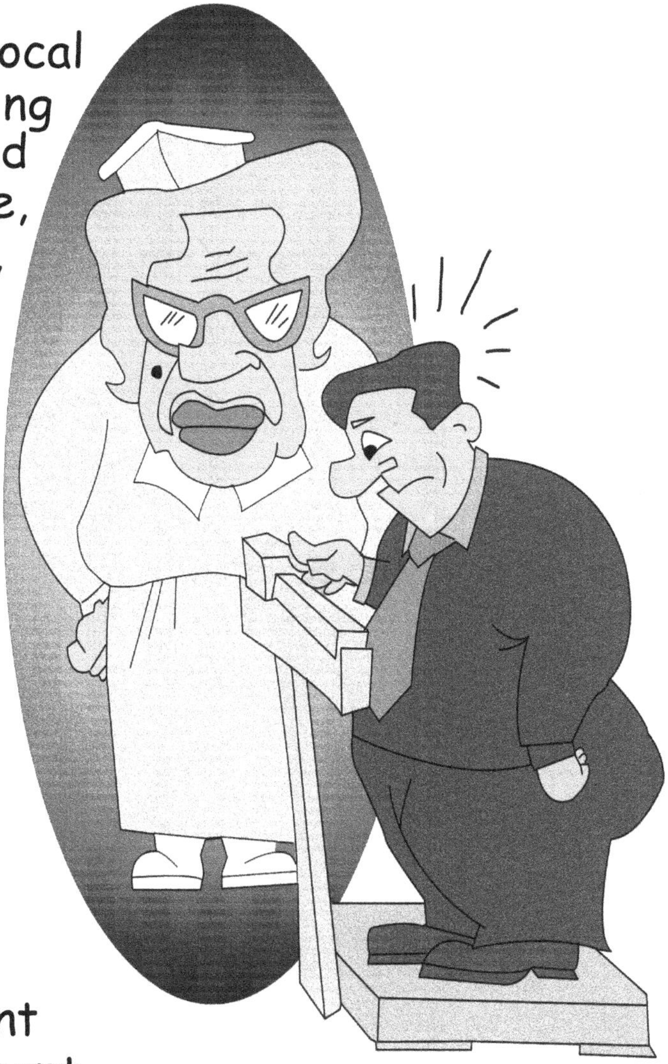

Last December I visited a local medical clinic. The first thing that nosey Nurse Beotche did was make me step on a scale, then announced to the world, **"265 pounds!"**

Holy crap, I'm getting pissed all over again just thinking about Nurse Beotche's arrogant attitude.

For a man six feet tall and weighing in at 265 pounds, the only way to look half-ass decent is to do some Hasslehoffing. We've all done it—sucked in that gut!

But Nurse Beotch fired me up and told me about Sergeant Otto. I thought, "WTF, Sergeant Otto? Here is a lamebrain with a name you can spell forwards or backwards and still get it right! What can he teach me about anything…?"

In my first meeting with Sergeant Otto, he reminded me that the scale goes below 200—not starts at 200!

Exercise? Not for me. Exercise makes me hungry! Eat a balanced diet? Maybe, but for now who freakin' cares! I just wanted to get my weight and blood pressure in the normal range!

"You can incorporate an exercise routine and a balanced diet into your new habits to maintain your weight **after** you reach your goal," I told myself, "that's how ya' roll."

Have you watched the GEICO commercial on TV with the drill sergeant therapist? Remember the opening bunkhouse scene with the new recruits and the drill sergeant in the movie *Full Metal Jacket*? Seen the Tide commercial with the drill sergeant who was angry about the dirty spot on the military uniform? All great stuff and easy to find and watch.

"YOU-TUBE ALL THREE OF THESE — DO IT NOW!"

"WE'LL WAIT ON YA, DICKWAD!"

"You back, TUBBY? You like those videos? Then carry on."

The DRILL SERGEANT CREED: ***"I will assist each individual in his efforts to become well disciplined...and I will instill pride!"***

Meet your personal instructor, **Drill Sergeant OTTO KLUTCH**. He's in-your-face and overbearing. He has the maturity of a fifteen-year-old, the testosterone level of a twenty-one-year-old, and the wisdom of a forty-five-year-old, all rolled into one nasty SOB!

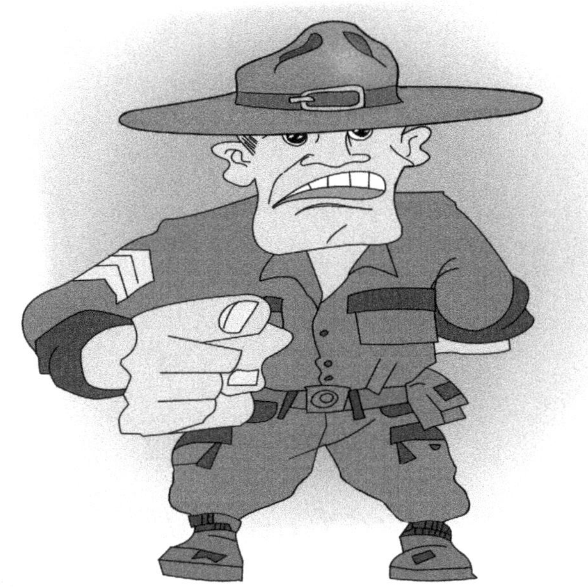

"I, Sergeant Otto, will be up your rectum, ya' freakin' pantywaist!"

"NO MORE EXCUSES—I WILL TEAR YOU A NEW ONE. BALLS TO THE WALL, BABY! WE ARE GOING TO CHANGE YOUR EATING HABITS!"

"YOU WILL LOSE THAT GUT!
SUCK IT UP, GIVE ME 20, DOUCHEBAG!"

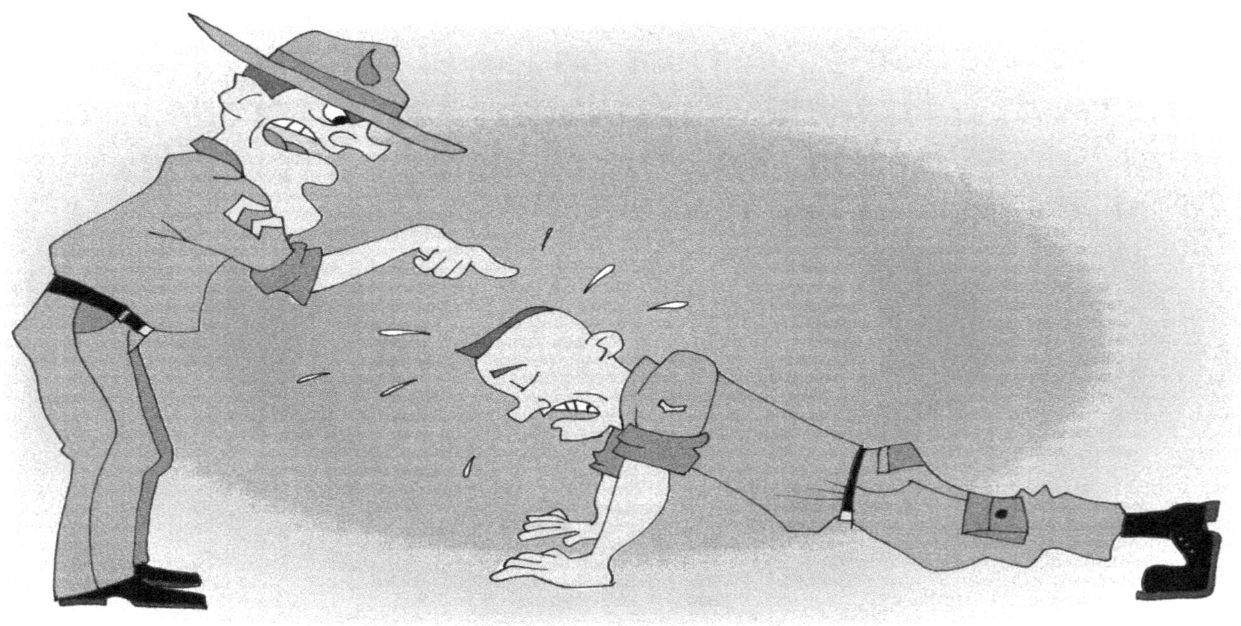

"You wouldn't have picked up this manual if you didn't need to lose a few pounds, LARDO."

"SO WHO'S YOUR DADDY NOW, NUMBNUTS?"

Sergeant Otto is going to play a little 'kick-ass' and teach you how to lose that weight and keep it off.

"You will enjoy what you eat MORE THAN EVER while you change your eating habits!"

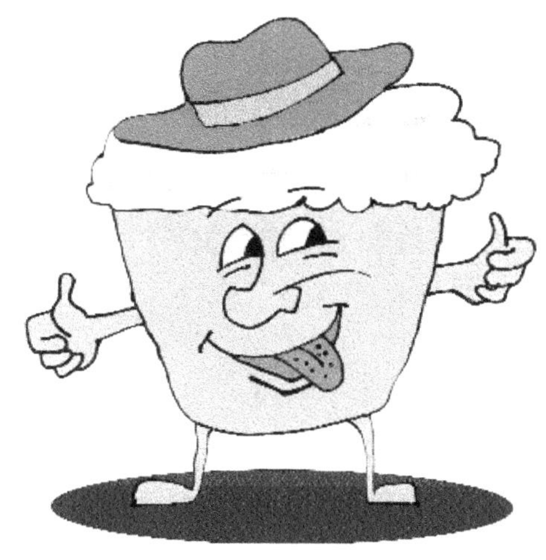

"Now look, CUPCAKE."

Maybe you thought about trying one of those "girly" weight loss food programs. You know the names. Unless you are blind, you had to see the disclaimer—results not typical!

Well then, what is typical? Advertisements and sales of programs that produce yo-yo weight loss.

"You got time for that, MISS PIGGY?"

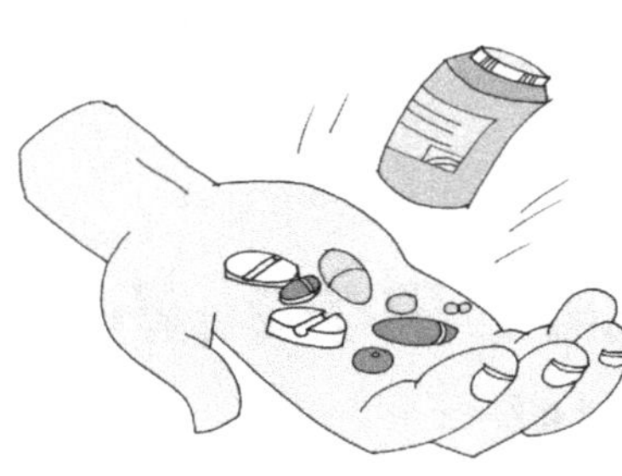

How about over-the-counter medication and prescription weight loss pills? Don't take my word for it.

"GOOGLE IT, A-HOLE!"

"What did you find? Worthless—that's what!"

Do you want to see a **fat** doctor? Do you know the risks of surgery?

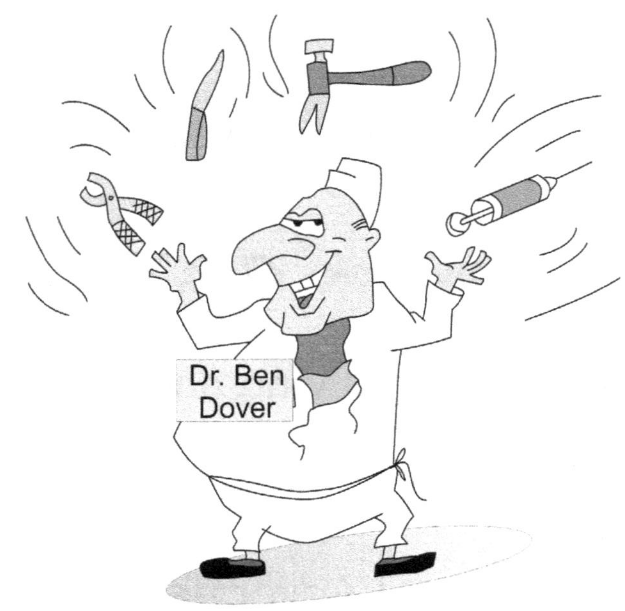

"GOOGLE THE COSTS OF THOSE OPTIONS, MORON!"

"Let's not 'waist' more of your time!"

"I WILL DRILL NEW EATING HABITS INTO YOUR FREAKIN' SKULL, PISSANT!"

"YOU WILL MAKE BETTER CHOICES USING *Sergeant Otto Man Diet*."

"Wanna cure your lack-a-nookie?"

"Wanna stay a fatso or trim up?"

"NOW IS YOUR CHANCE TO LOSE RATHER THAN STAY A BUBBLEBUTT LOSER!"

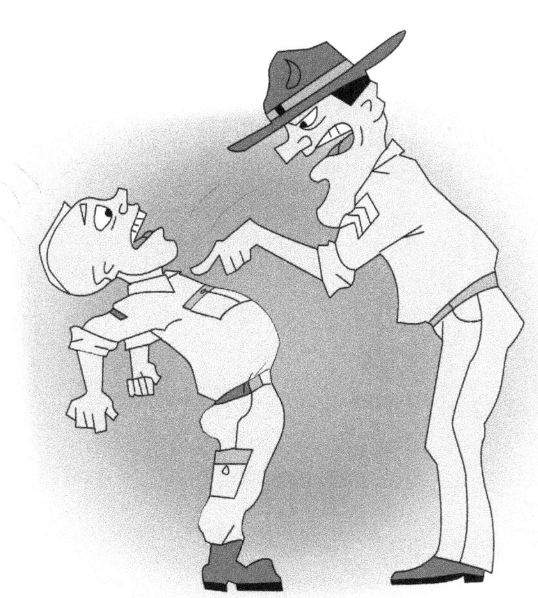

"YOU READY FOR THIS? LET'S GET AFTER IT!"

"GOT GONADS?"

Chapter 2

Mantra Time, not Miller Time—
LARDASS!

"Hey you, JUMBO! Tell me, what is a mantra? Is it a repetitive phrase, slogan, chant?"

"SIR, YES, SIR!"

Try 80 by 8. That was my New Year's resolution—80 pounds by my birthday in August—8 months. Yeah, sure! And just like every year, I promise to lose weight, save money, exercise more, work smarter.

But whoa! I did it—lost the 80 pounds one month early—July. **Sa-weeeet!** Why this year and never before? Sergeant Otto and his instructions, that's why!

First: Sergeant Otto made me set a goal—80 pounds.
Second: Sergeant Otto made me set a deadline—my birthday in eight months—August. The formula 80 by 8, 80x8.

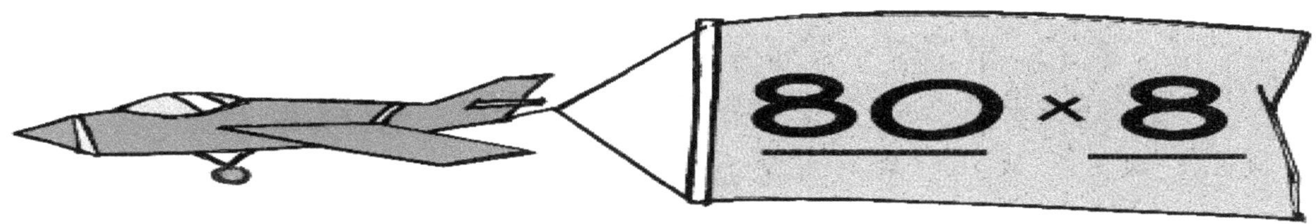

First time I had ever been specific about weight loss. Before Sergeant Otto, I just wanted to "lose a few."

"GO GET A PEN, MAGGOT! NO MORE READING TILL YOU PICK UP A PEN!"

"You ready now, SWEETHEART?"

Here are a few suggestions. Wanna lose 2 pants sizes in 2 months? Try 2x2. Getting married in 6 months and want to lose 30 pounds? How about 30x6?

"How much do you want to lose and when do you want to reach your goal, CREAMPUFF?"

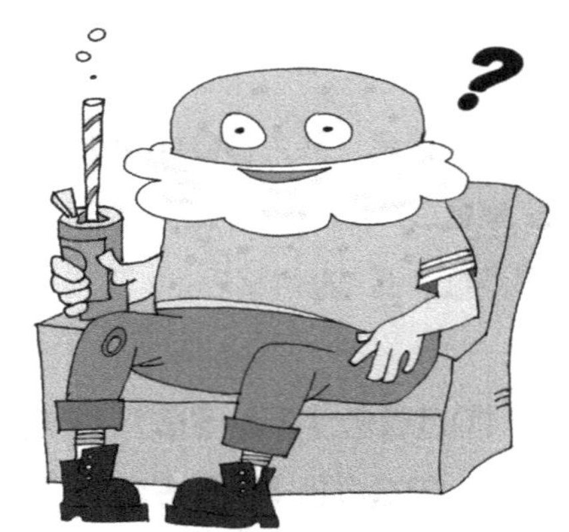

"THINK HARD, PUTZ!"

"NO MORE 'DRY-HUMPING' DIETS. INSTEAD, THIS TIME YOU WILL GET RESULTS!"

"You will repeat your mantra to yourself before you go to bed, when you wake-up, before you eat, when driving, when walking—constantly!"

"Time to start your loss, HOSS!
This is important crap.
YOU WILL NOT FAIL AGAIN."

Two pounds a week is 8 to 10 pounds a month, 50 freakin'-pounds in 6 months, 100 pounds in a year!

"Ok, EINSTEIN—ya' got it?
Need help with your mantra?"

"DO ONE THING ON YOUR OWN
IN YOUR PATHETIC LIFE!"

"COMMIT NOW! GROW UP, NUTSACK!"

"DON'T GO ANUS-THE-MENACE ON ME!"

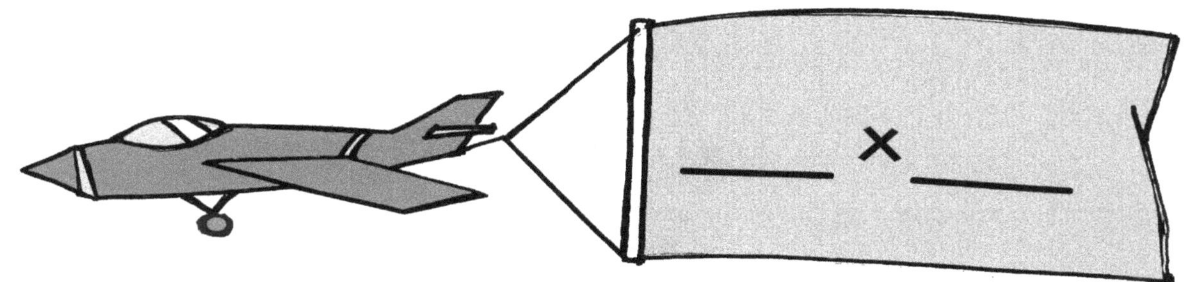

"JUST WRITE YOUR FREAKIN' MANTRA."

Now it's time to learn a new medical term: **carbories**. Carbories are the total of carbohydrates plus the calories in each food item we eat and drink.

Since **you are** a porker and **I was** a porker, I know neither of us are carb/calorie counters. Sergeant Otto will teach you how to "know" the carbories you eat every day. No research, no time commitment. It will become easy. That is a promise—just keep reading!

You will consider both carbs **and** calories in deciding how aggressive you want to be in your weight loss. Seventeen hundred carbories (1625 calories and 75 carbs per day) will produce consistent weight loss. Better yet, 1250 carbories (1200 calories and 50 carbs per day) will produce accelerated weight loss. You will dump the pounds **FAST!**

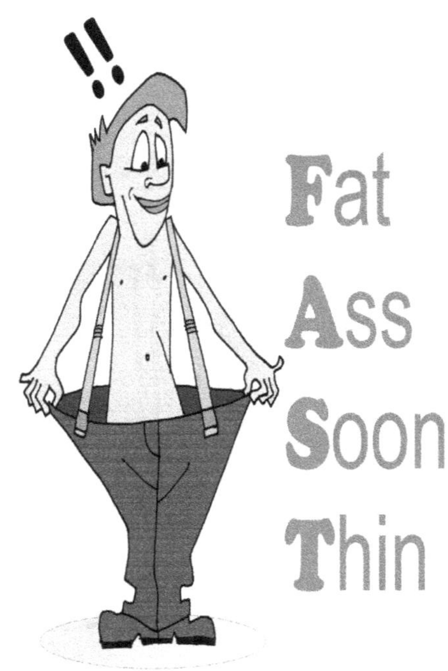

Look at your mantra again—is it realistic? Are you setting yourself up to fail? Want to change it?

Now, 80x8 is me. **What are you?** About 1250 carbories a day got me to my goal a month early. Think about your mantra! All you need is a pen and a pledge.

"SCREAM IT FROM THE ROOFTOPS!"

"Is it a realistic goal?"

"WRITE IT AGAIN, BUTTWIPE!"

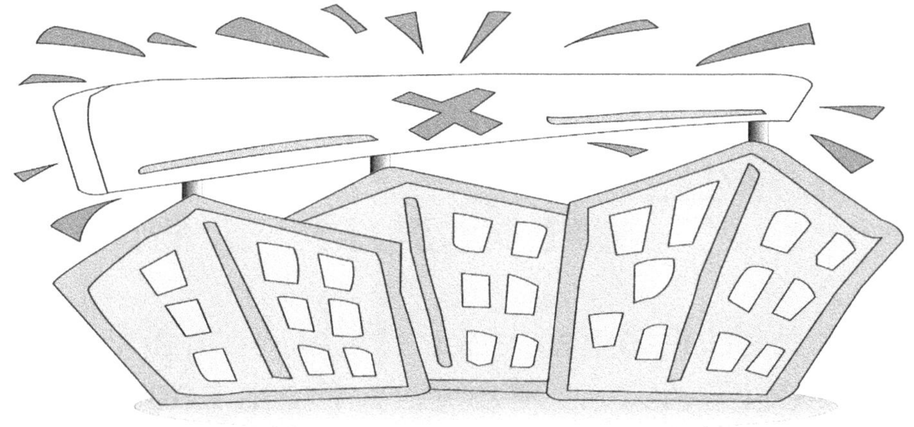

You better have written your mantra by now or Sergeant Otto will kick your slimy, sleazy....

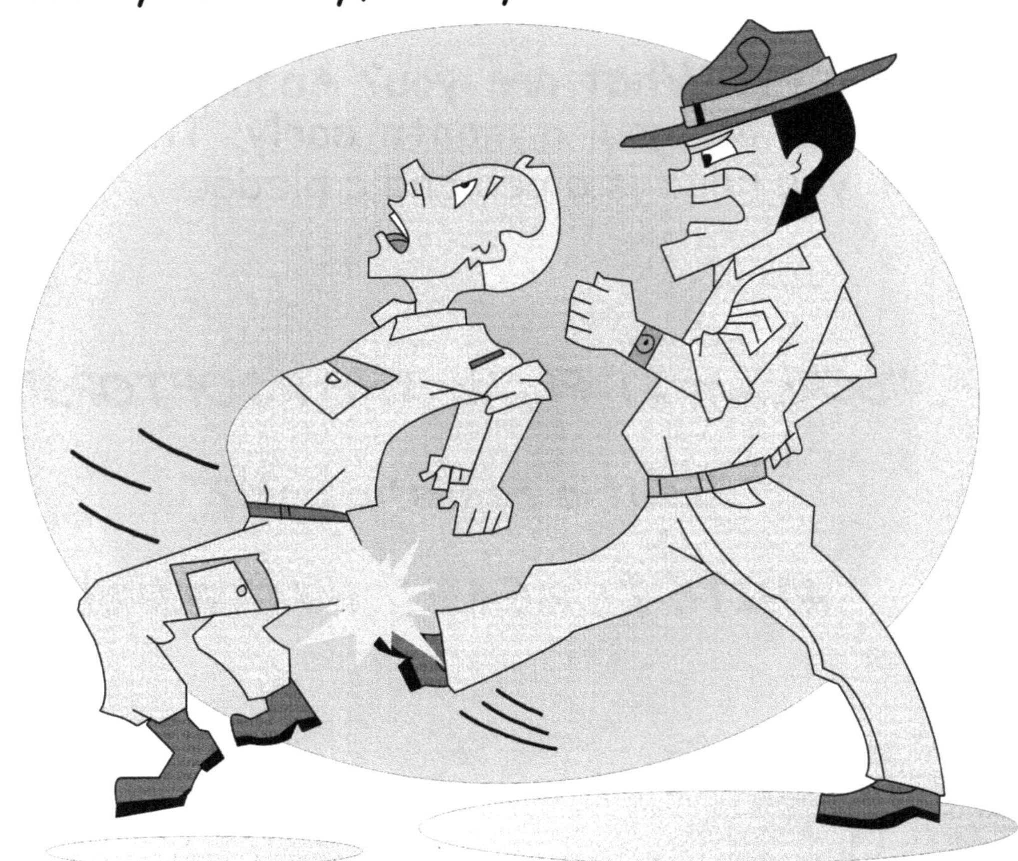

"YOU WILL BE THANKING ME LATER, CRISCOBUTT!"

Now we are getting somewhere. Feel better? Take a break. "It's Miller time." Have a beer and think about this new commitment to yourself.

"In the rest of this manual I will show you how to reach your goal—proud of you so far, CHUBS."

"HOWEVER, IF YOU THINK THIS HAS BEEN A STUPID ASSIGNMENT, THEN THROW THIS MANUAL IN THE TRASH, SWEAT HOG!"

Call Sergeant Otto and you will get a refund of your money.

The phone number is...

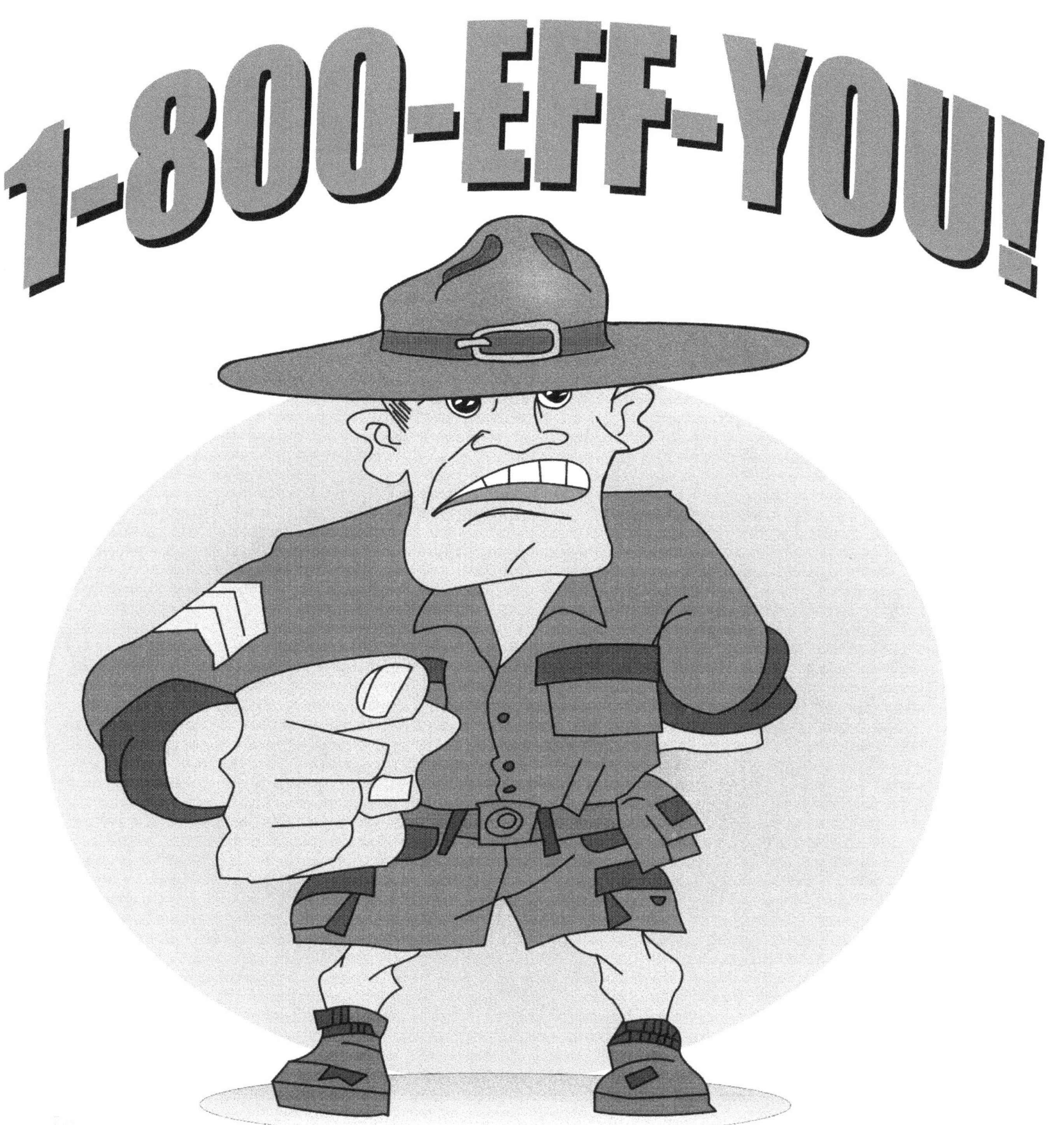
1-800-EFF-YOU!

Chapter 3

Variety is the VICE of Life

"Who can YOU blame for your fat gut?"

Hey man, you are reading this because you need to shrink your gut. But many of us have convinced ourselves that our weight problem is someone else's fault. Think back. Who was in charge of the house when you were growing up?

"YER MOMMA!"

Right or wrong—around the house momma's rules were law!

When you were a kid, did you ever hear something similar to this? "Do not wear the same clothes two days in a row—you wore those things yesterday!"

"Your momma isn't looking over your shoulder anymore. But do ya' wear the same clothes on Tuesday that you wore on Monday?"

We both know the answer to that bone-headed question!

That same *'MomPhilosophy'* applied by mothers to meal preparation produced two god-awful adult eating habits!

FIRST: Can you hear her now? "We had that for lunch—find something else." And remember this one? "NO! We had that for dinner last night..."

"Does this ring a bell, JERKFACE?"

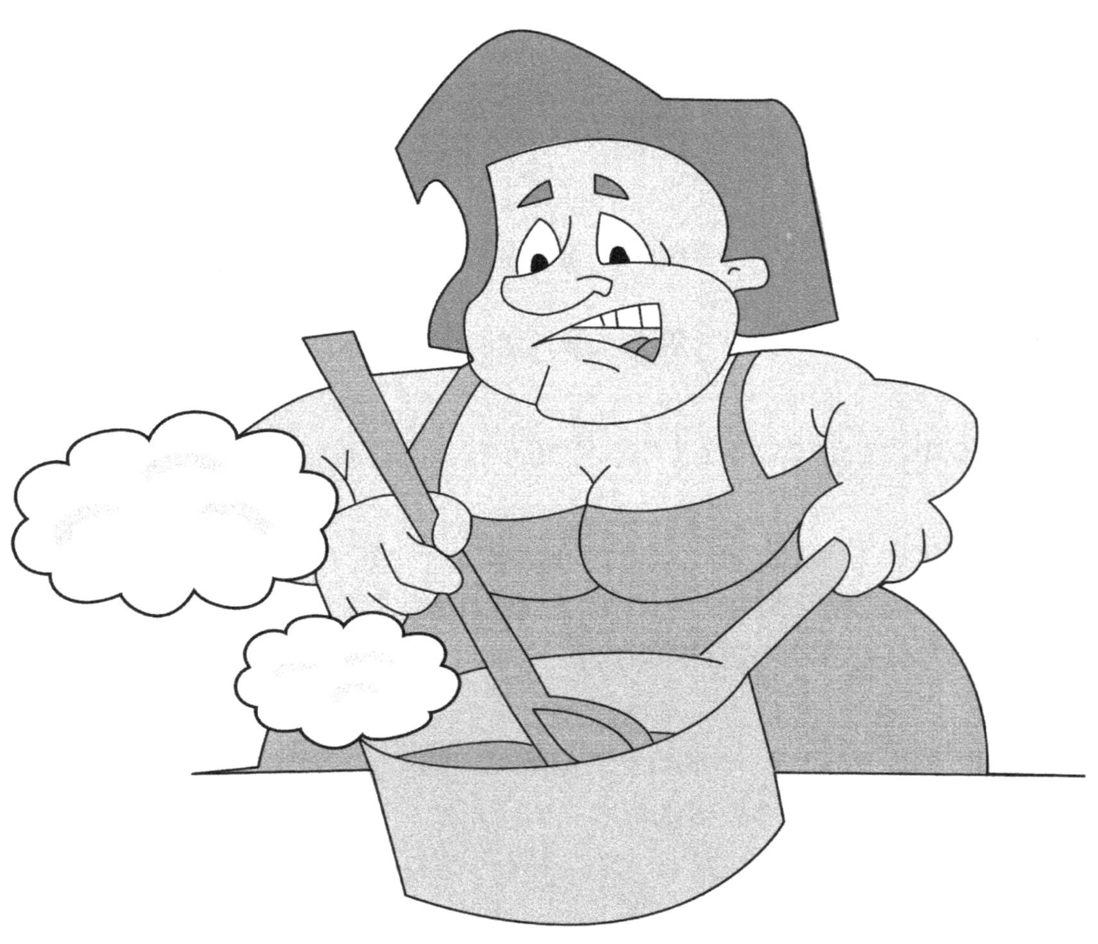

"Good ole mom. Gettin' ready to bust your chops."

SECOND: How can you forget?

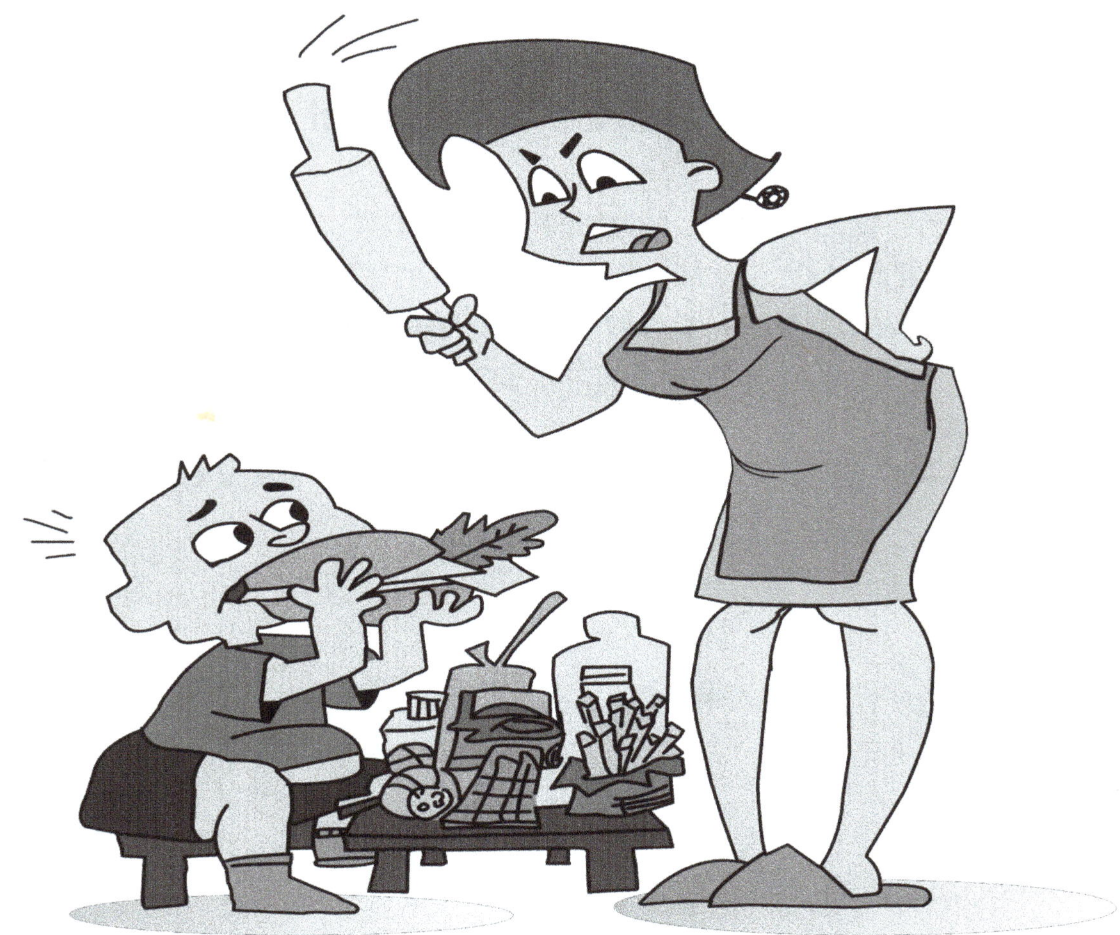

"You are not leaving until your **plate is empty, BUSTER!"**

It definitely didn't matter if you liked the food or if the food was healthy and good for you.

The only concern was that you "gobbled" **all** of the variety of foods prepared by momma!

Mommas taught the **more variety** rules: 1. Constantly changing clothes. 2. Making sure that what you eat today was different from what you ate yesterday. 3. Forced eating of all the variety of foods prepared for a meal by your momma.

"When did this 'variety is the spice of life' bull crap start? I love your momma, but she didn't teach you squat about the secrets of weight control!"

"YO—I'M TALKING TO YOU, PORKCHOP!"

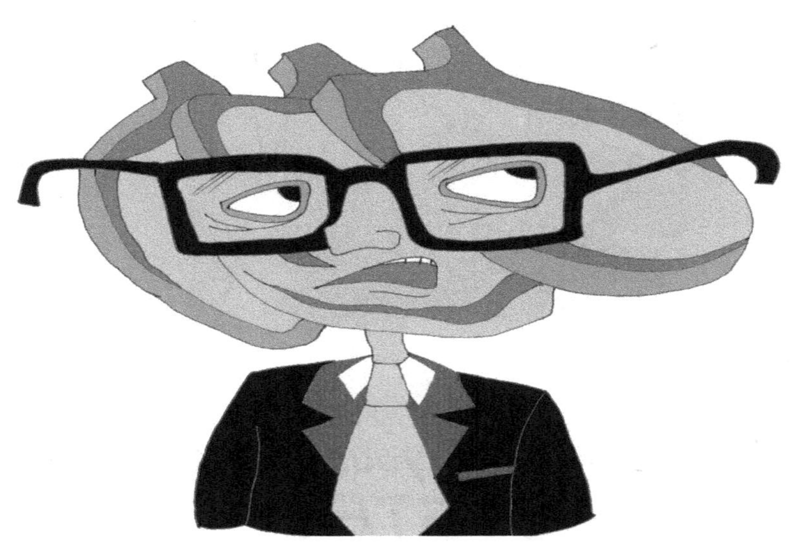

"Your momma got it bass ackwards, DILDO."

"The truth is...
VARIETY IS THE VICE OF LIFE."

You **can** eat the same thing for lunch and dinner—and love it. You **can** eat the same thing for dinner two, three, four nights in a row—and love it. And you definitely do not need to eat all of the prepared food all of the time.

"LEFTOVERS is not a four-letter word."

This need for **variety** taught by your momma is one of the causes of weight problems and one of the reasons you are reading this manual.

"SCREAM IT NOW, OINKER!"

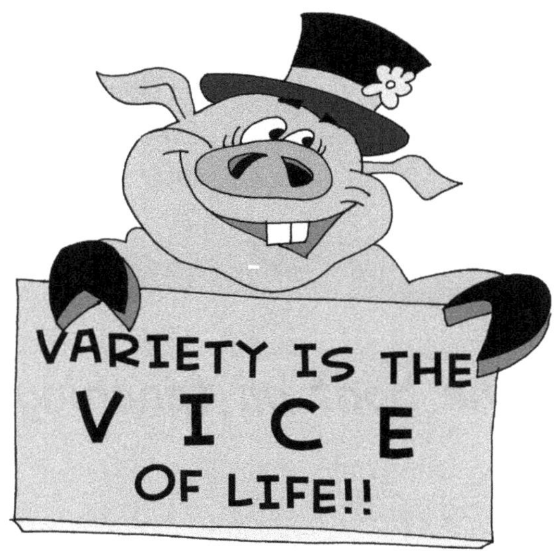

"You are going to learn how you can reduce the variety of foods you eat, reduce your gut, and enjoy eating more than ever, PORKY."

Your momma was right about a lot of things, damn straight! She taught you the difference between a windbreaker and breaking wind, didn't she?

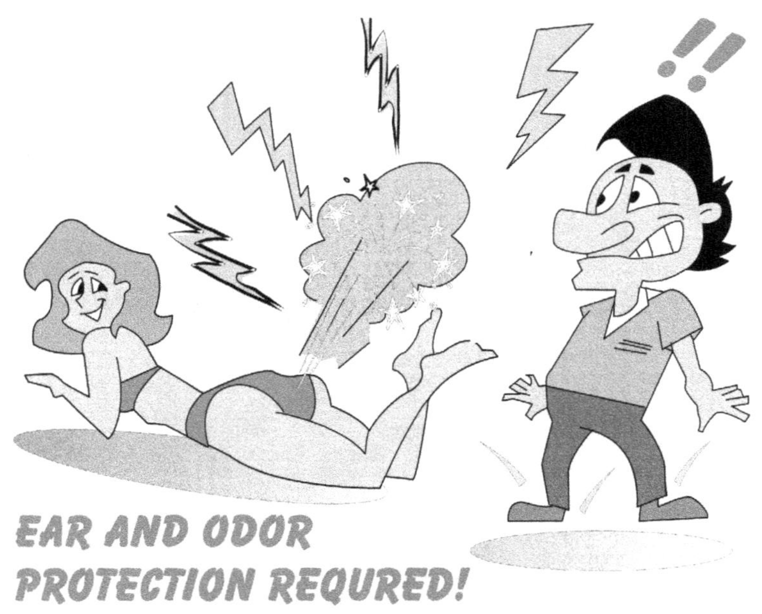

"But she missed the boat on teaching weight control."

You decide...

"Do you want to be EYE-CANDY or I-CHUBBY?"

"WHAT'S YOUR MANTRA?"

"WRITE IT BELOW."

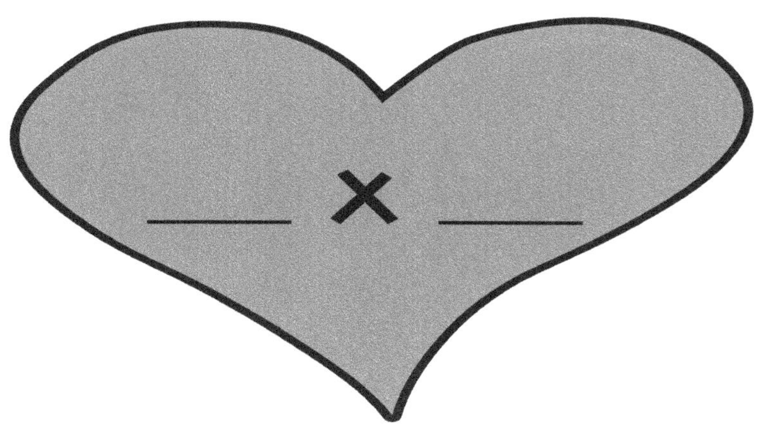

"VARIETY IS THE VICE OF LIFE.
SAY IT!"

"GOT IT SO FAR, WUSSY?"

Chapter 4

Love It or Leave It!

"NOW SIT UP STRAIGHT, FATASS!"

So how are you going to reduce the variety of food you eat and enjoy eating more?

"LISTEN UP, GOMER!"

We eat foods we love, foods we like, and some foods that are just ok.

But if you eat and drink junk you don't like, you need more help than Sergeant Otto can give you!

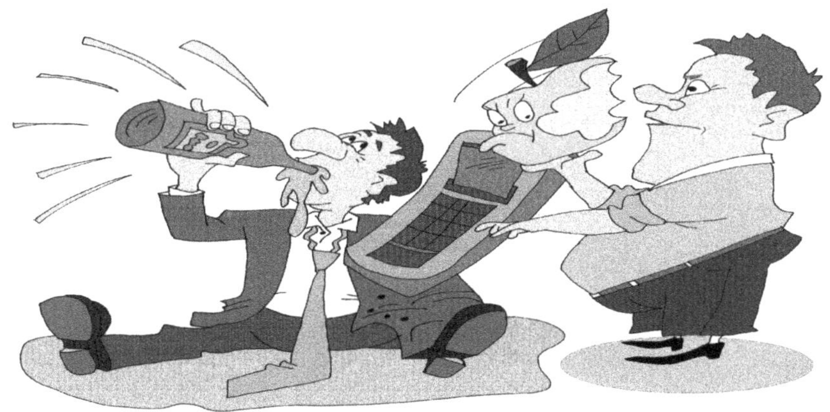

"CALL A THERAPIST, BUTTHOLE!"

Do each of the written exercises that follow. The writing assignments will force you to focus on everything that you cram down your pie-hole! You will learn to monitor the quantity of food you choose to eat that keeps you overweight. And you will start separating the healthy things that you love to eat from your less healthy choices.

"This is not food torture, soldier!"

"Got your pen, HUGH-JAZZ?"

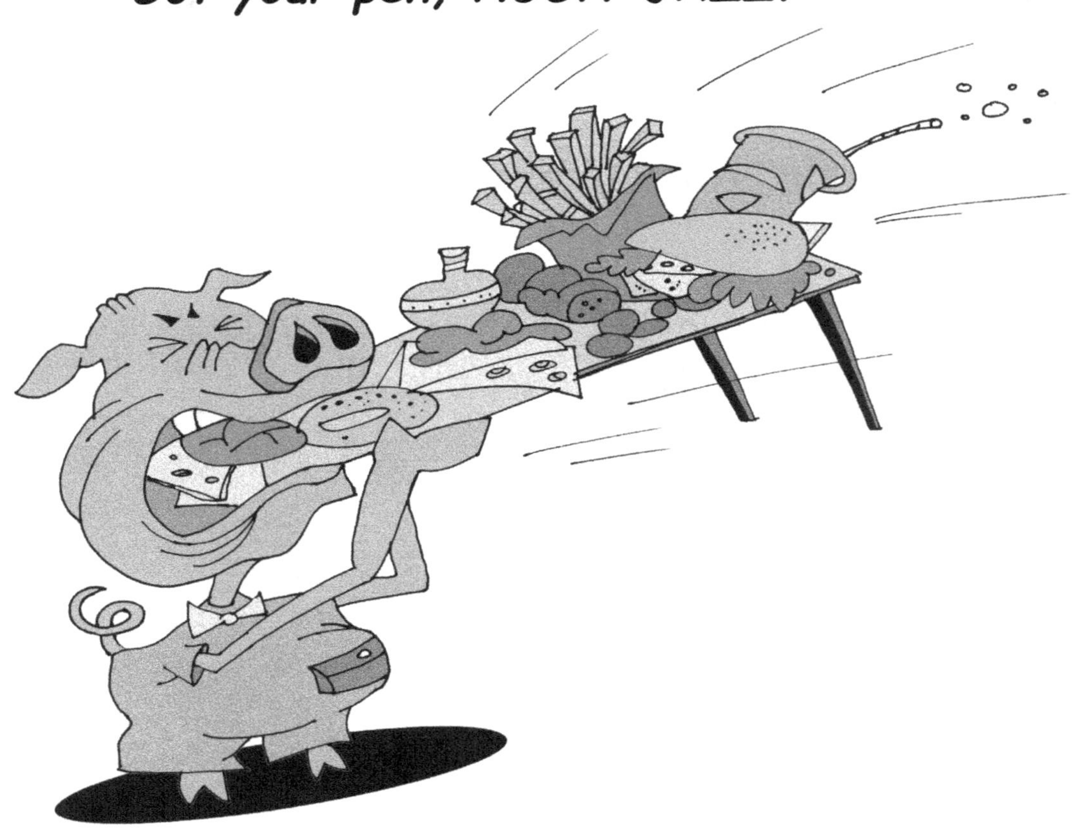

"AAUUUGGHHH, GULP!"

Step 1. You will make a list of the foods that you love to eat—your FAVES. Don't separate healthy, sugars, good, bad, fattening. If necessary, get a separate piece of paper to list your favorite foods.

"If you love it, you write it, SCUMBAG!"

YOUR FAVES

______________________	______________________
______________________	______________________
______________________	______________________
______________________	______________________
______________________	______________________
______________________	______________________
______________________	______________________

Think of all the breakfasts, lunches, snacks, and dinners you love—your yummies...your FAVES.

"IF YOU DON'T LOVE IT, THEN LEAVE IT OFF YOUR LIST, DUMBASS!"

"DONE? I SAID—ARE YOU FREAKIN' DONE?"

"IS YOUR LIST OF FAVES COMPLETE?"

Step 2. Unless you live in a cave, you **know** the things that you **should** eat regularly and the things you **should** eat only occasionally or not at all.

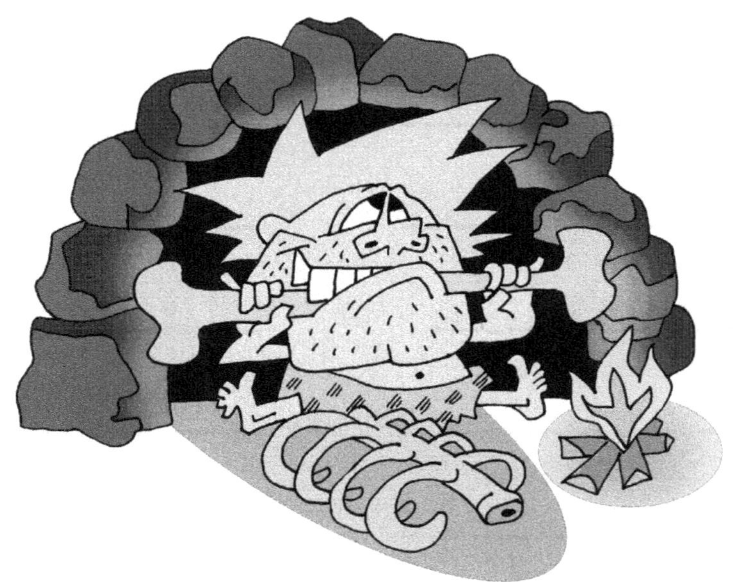

"NOW LOOK AT YOUR LIST OF FAVES, YA' JERKOFF!"

To achieve your goal, you are going to pick what you **should** eat from your personal list of FAVES that you just completed on the previous page!

"You may not have a ton of variety, but you will only be eating the foods you love!"

You're going to search your list and find lower carborie foods (see page 12) that are **also** the foods you love to eat! It's easy! Chicken, fish, meat, fruit, veggies, and eggs are a few suggestions—do some research—check Atkins, Weight Watchers, Jenny Craig, Dr. Joel Fuhrman, and others.

"What do you love to eat with low carbories, BLUBBERBUTT?"

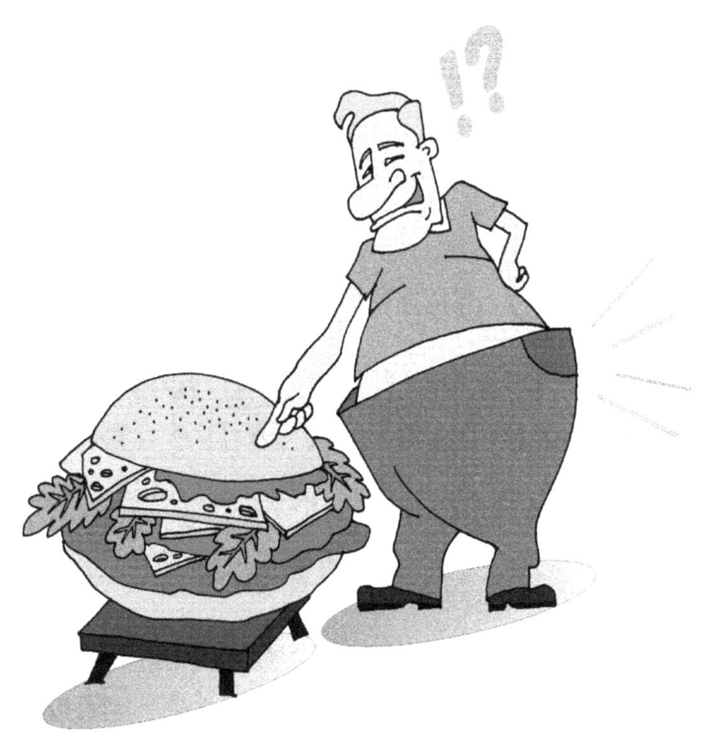

"START WRITING, HUMUNGO."

"Now make a short list below from your original list of FAVES."

YOUR LIST OF LOW CARBORIE FAVES	

"YOU GET IT, D-BAG?"

"You need to start eating low carbories. But only what you love OR leave it off your list!"

"REMEMBER—VARIETY IS THE VICE OF LIFE."

"Variety got you where you are today! Do you want variety or a 34-inch waist?"

"The good news? This 'reduced variety' habit— IT IS ONLY TEMPORARY."

Once you hit your goal, add back higher carborie foods and establish a balanced diet. If you gain a few pounds—then get back to your menu of low carbories for a week or two. And guess what—all the time you are only eating the foods you love—your FAVES.

"Come on, how easy is that?"

"YOU MADE YOUR LIST, BUTTERBALL?"

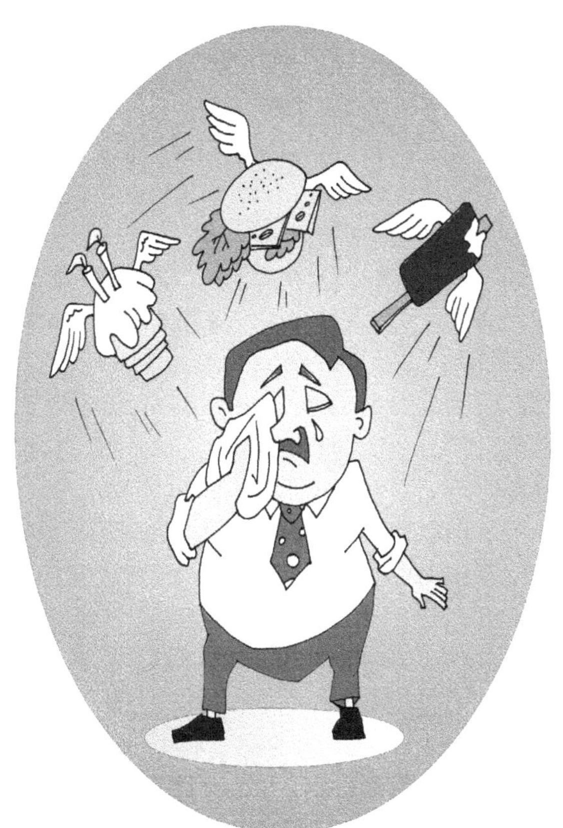

"DON'T BE A WIMPY CRYBABY—MAN UP!"

Step 3. You need to take your list of low carborie foods that you love from step 2 and make a weekly menu. Check out my menu on page 69.

"Fill in your weekly menu now, DOUGH-BOY."

YOUR WEEKLY MENU

	M	T	W	Th	F	S	S
Breakfast							
Lunch							
Snack							
Dinner							
Dessert							

"Put your menu on a separate piece of paper, DUMBO."

Step 4. In the last chapter you will also find my list of low carborie snacks and meal substitutions used to compliment my daily menu. Use mine as a guideline. This is the final step.

YOUR LIST OF LOW CARBORIE SNACKS
AND MEAL COMPLIMENT FAVES

______________________	______________________
______________________	______________________
______________________	______________________
______________________	______________________

"EASY—JUST REPEAT YOUR WEEKLY MENU UNTIL YOU REACH YOUR GOAL, THUNDER THIGHS!"

"When you hit your target, then you can get back to selecting a larger variety of foods!"

"Eat the same low carborie foods two-three times a day, IF YOU LOVE IT."

"Eat the same thing for lunch every day, IF YOU LOVE IT."

"Eat the same low carborie dinners and snacks every day, IF YOU LOVE IT."

"FOLLOW THE INSTRUCTIONS BELOW, SCHMUCK!"

1. **Write** your mantra:

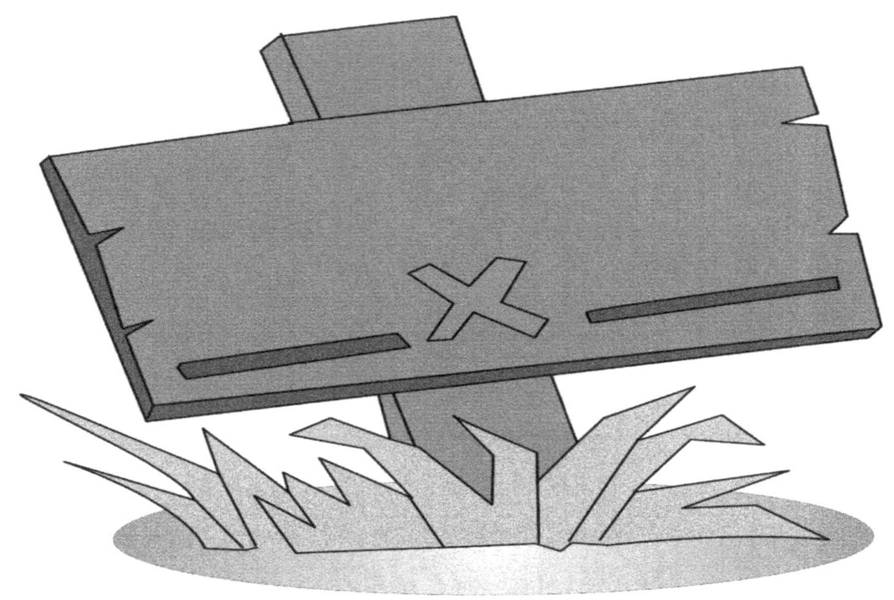

2. **Say it:** "Variety is the ________(blank)________ of life!"

3. **Say it:** "Love it or ________(blank)________ it!"

"You, a JACKOFFICER, are now armed with your FAVES weekly menu and list of low carborie snacks."

"Using <u>Sergeant Otto Man Diet</u>, you will declare war and attack the one remaining problem…."

Chapter 5

Slip Happens!

"HELLO, we are not perfect eaters—SLIP HAPPENS!"

You know what you should eat, and now you have made the decision to confront the enemy—food temptations.

"Get combat ready to minimize poor eating choices—time to engage the three primary causes of SLIP HAPPENS!"

The first threat is media advertising—TV, newspaper, signs. Burger, pizza, and beer ads—food, constantly in your face.

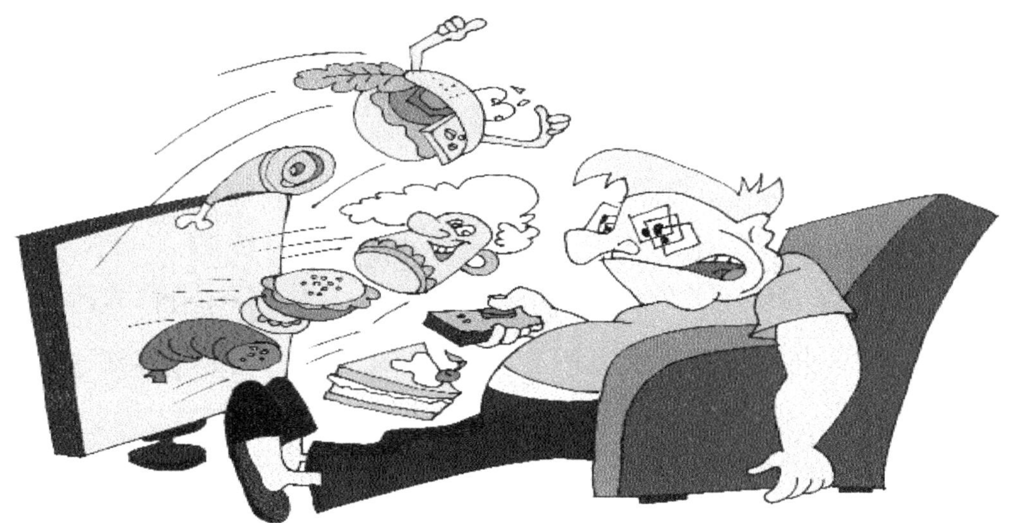

"Your weekly FAVES menu you created is now your weapon to fight temptations."

Your FAVES menu is the artillery to assist making good food selections. Keep it with you at all times.

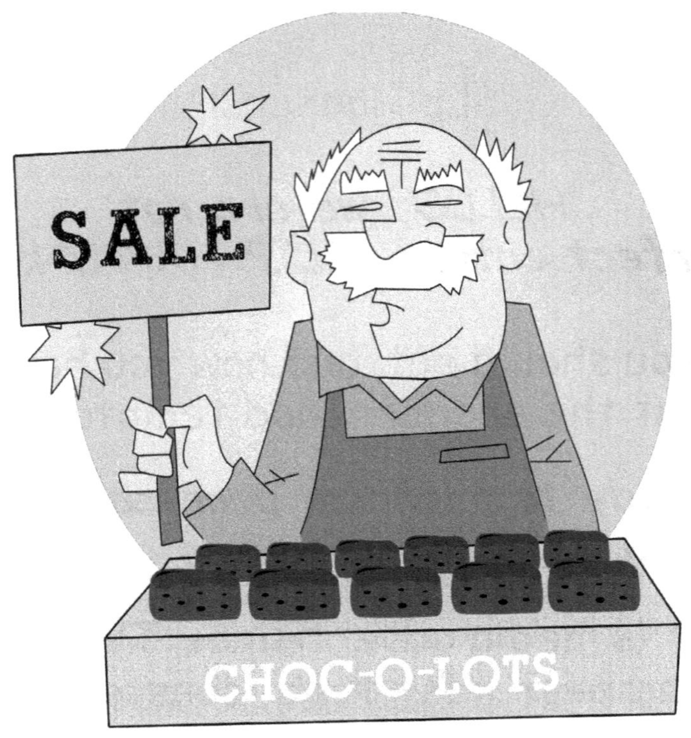

"Use your weekly FAVES menu to eliminate the threat of the 'MediaEnemy'."

The second battle is your assault on our childhood language training—"Food-Speak". It is a subtle and effective contributor to SLIP HAPPENS. We were taught "Food-Speak" starting when we were very young. It happened to us and now we blindly teach it to our kids!

"Listen up—I don't want to hear that 'NOT ME' crap!"

Ever heard or said "Joe Blow **went bananas**?" WENT BANANAS? You got to be kiddin' me! Did you ever see someone morph by losing their arms, legs, face, and then turn bright yellow? I doubt it!

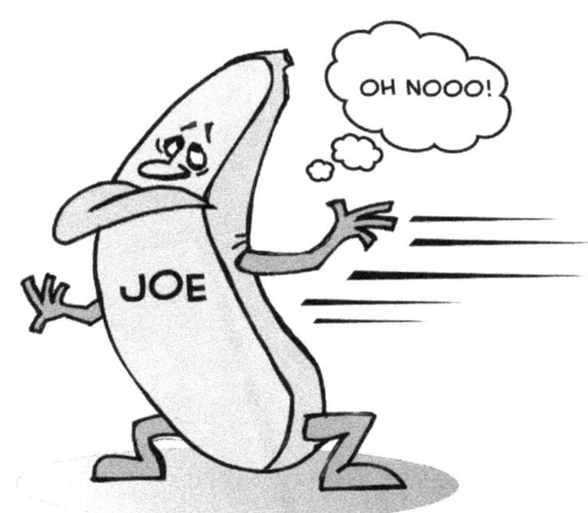

***"Joe may have gotten angry,
but he did NOT go bananas!"***

What about "blah, blah, blah is **food for thought!**" Here we go again. Imbedded in our mini-donkey-brains is the association of thinking with...FOOD! **Why?**

"Do you think Einstein was thinking about a peanut buster parfait from Dairy Queen while he was developing the theory of relativity, ASSWIPE?"

If the first thing that popped into your mind was that Dairy Queen probably wasn't around when Einstein was alive, then you have missed the point!

"Food-Speak" will eff you up. You are going to love this. Because of years of practice, playing the drums was a **piece... of...cake** for GutMan.

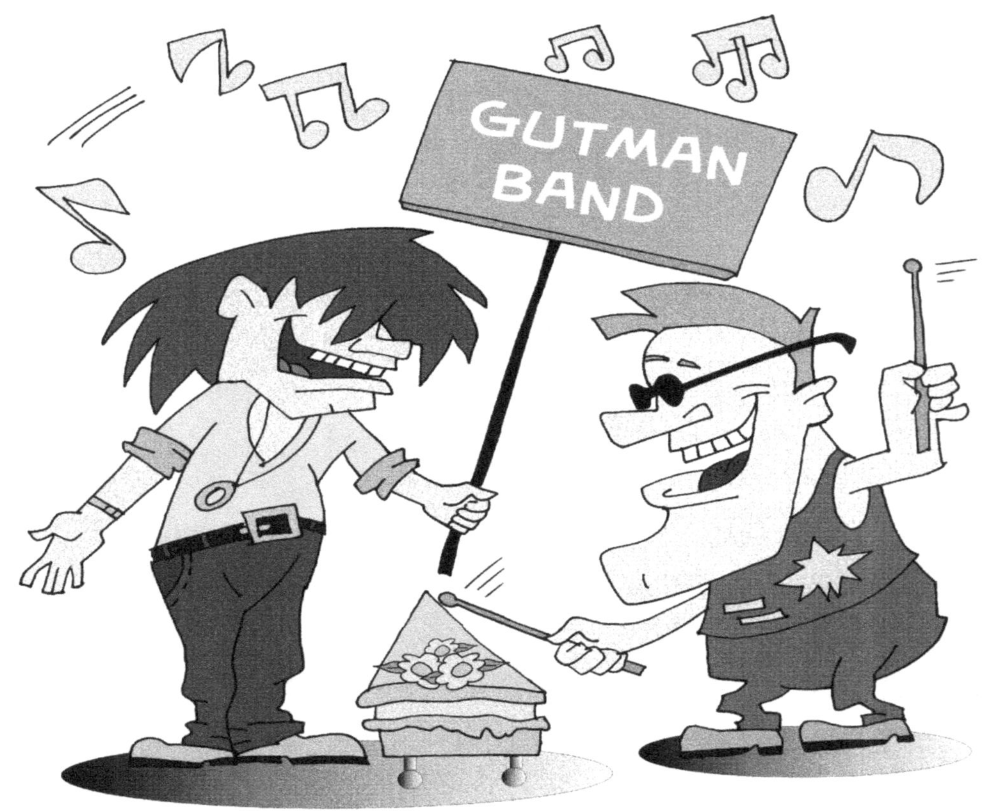

"A FREAKIN' PIECE...OF...CAKE?"

OMG...sad! Be sure and teach that one! We all learn this crap when young, then carry on the tradition. Without Sergeant Otto's help you do not have a chance. No surprise that you have a 42-inch waist!

"Get the idea, BUTTLOAD? Look at the last one."

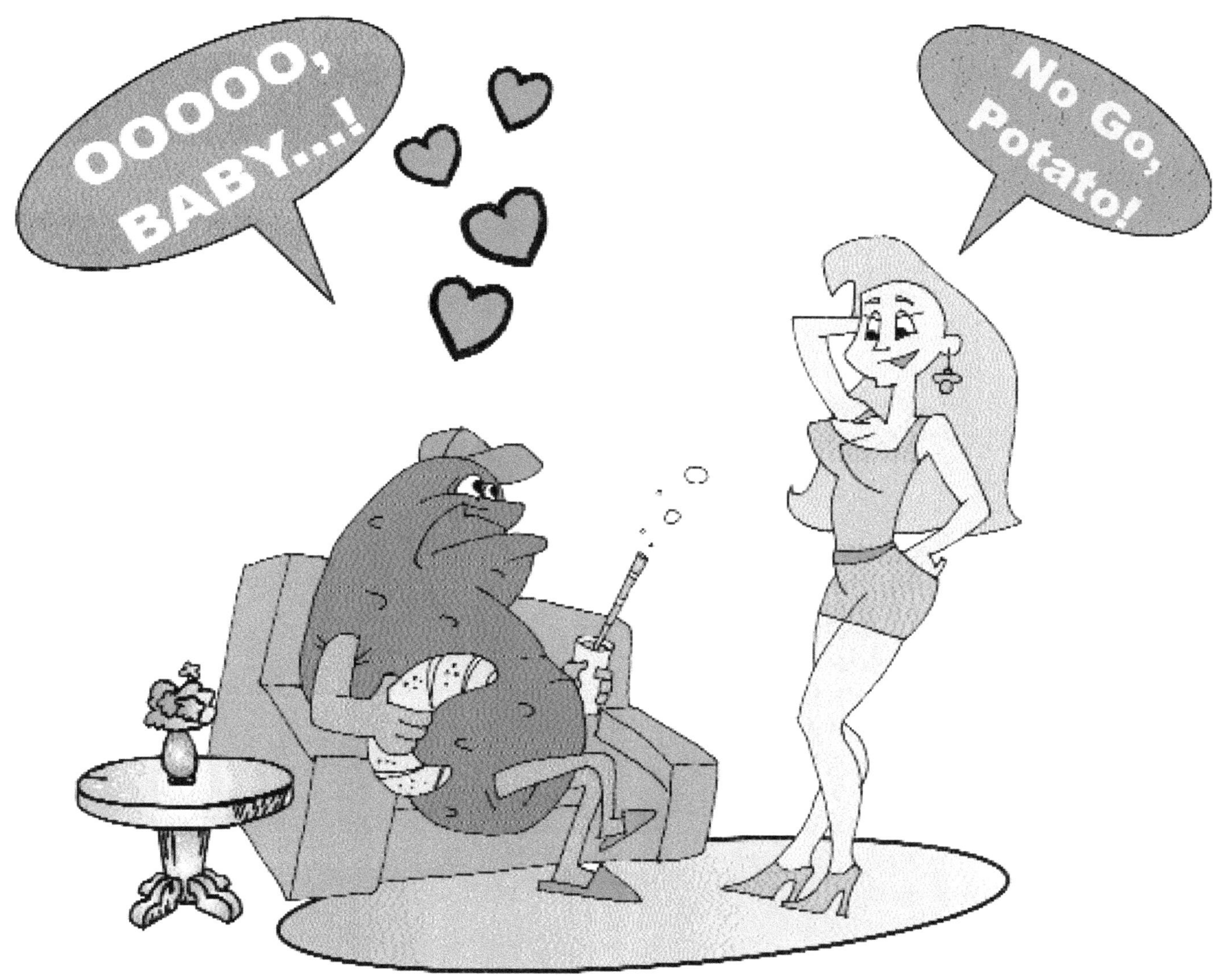

A bad day in the life of a...COUCH POTATO!

I'm sure you've heard "belly up, jam it in, veg out, eating away at me." If you know other "Food-Speak," send it to Sergeant Otto. Our language training is a subtle, constant, and under-cover food reminder contributing to SLIP HAPPENS!

Do Sergeant Otto a big favor—the next time you hear someone use "Food-Speak," send a clear message that we are not saying it anymore and we are not teaching it anymore! Then emphasize your point by giving them a big, quick, and hard...

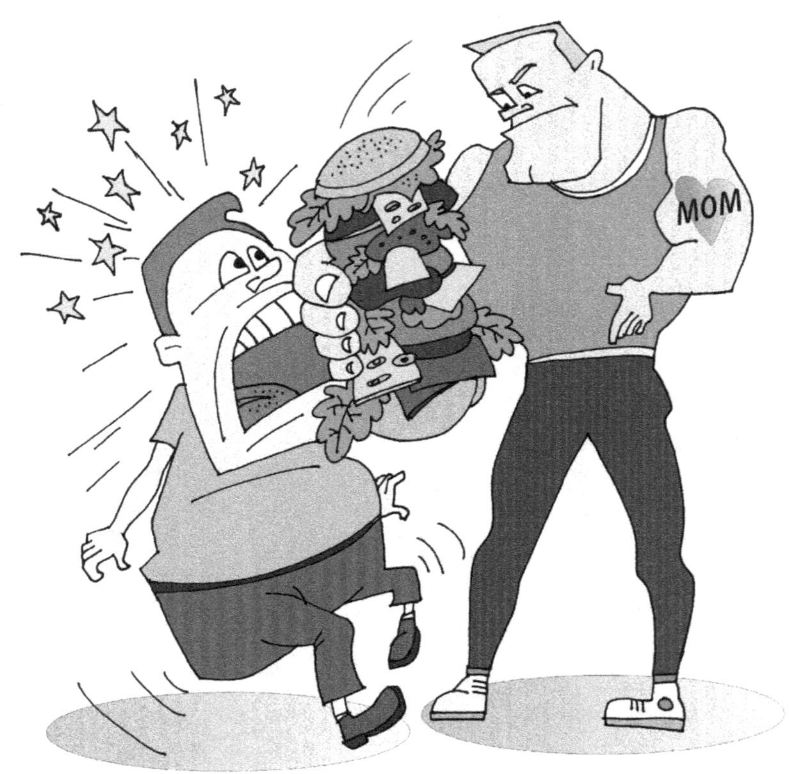

knuckle sandwich!

"WE DO NOT WANT TO BE CONSTANTLY THINKING AND TALKING ABOUT FOOD!"

"FIGHT 'FOOD-SPEAK'!"

The third and last conflict causing SLIP HAPPENS is social interaction. We both know what is coming...birthday, wedding, graduation, anniversary, retirement, vacation, holidays...the list is endless—all just waiting to ambush your plan!

What should you do to minimize "DietDamage" when you attend various social events? **Remember Noah?** It wasn't raining when Noah built the ark! **He planned ahead!** You need to do the same.

So what can you do **before** you attend these social events? Here are two suggestions: 1. Eat food from your menu before you leave home to help control your hunger. 2. Sneak in your own food that you listed on your FAVES menu.

You're smart, you're motivated—think of other ideas.

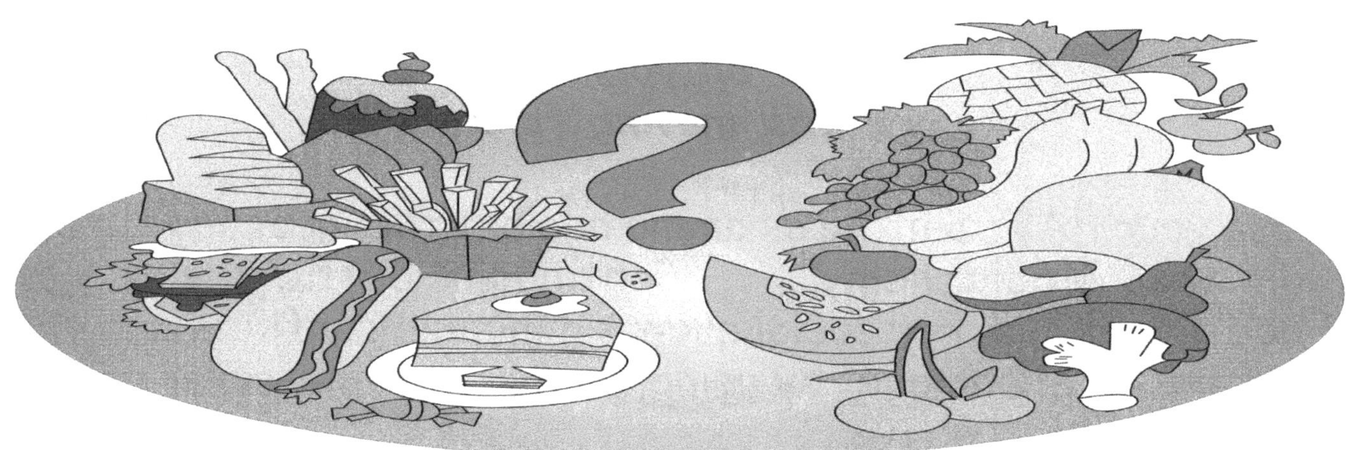

"Make your eating plan before it starts raining, NOAH!"

And then what should you do **after** you arrive? Eat only the items that you listed in your weekly menu of FAVES, substitutions, and snacks.

"This rule eliminates the junk!"

"JUST STICK TO YOUR MENU, SLEAZEBAG!"

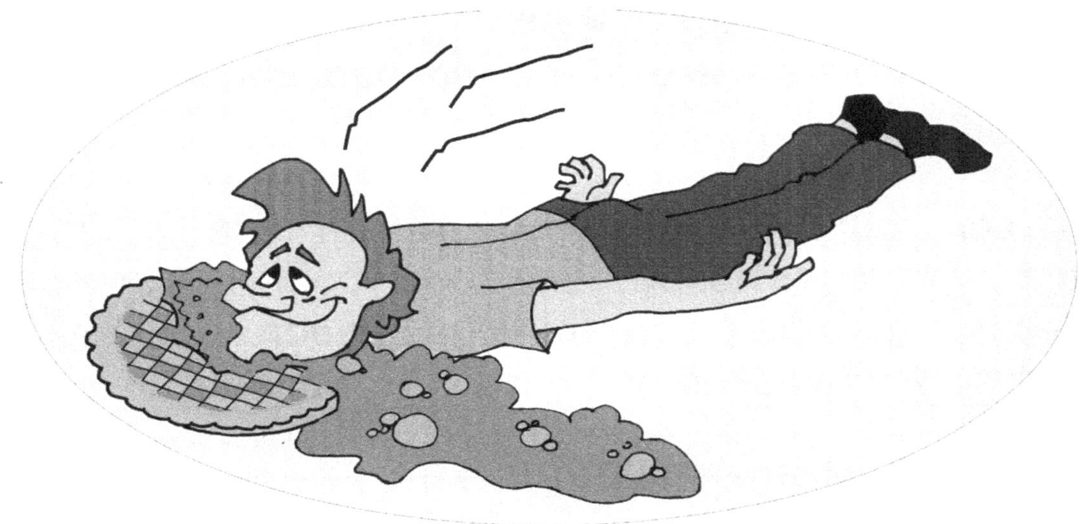

"But if you fall on your face, at least you are still moving forward."*

1. Use your FAVES menu as ammo against the incoming threat from the "MediaEnemy". 2. Continually battle the use of "Food-Speak". 3. For social events minimize conflicts and the resulting "DietDamage" by using the before-and-after eating guidelines listed above.

"You will conquer SLIP HAPPENS."

*Victor Kiam, New England Patriots

"Follow these rules with Sergeant Otto Man Diet and you will not suffer PREMATURE EXASPERATION."

"WHEN IT'S TIME FOR YOUR NEXT MEAL, JUST GET BACK TO YOUR FAVES MENU, QUEEFER!"

"SLIP HAPPENS, but tomorrow is another day!"

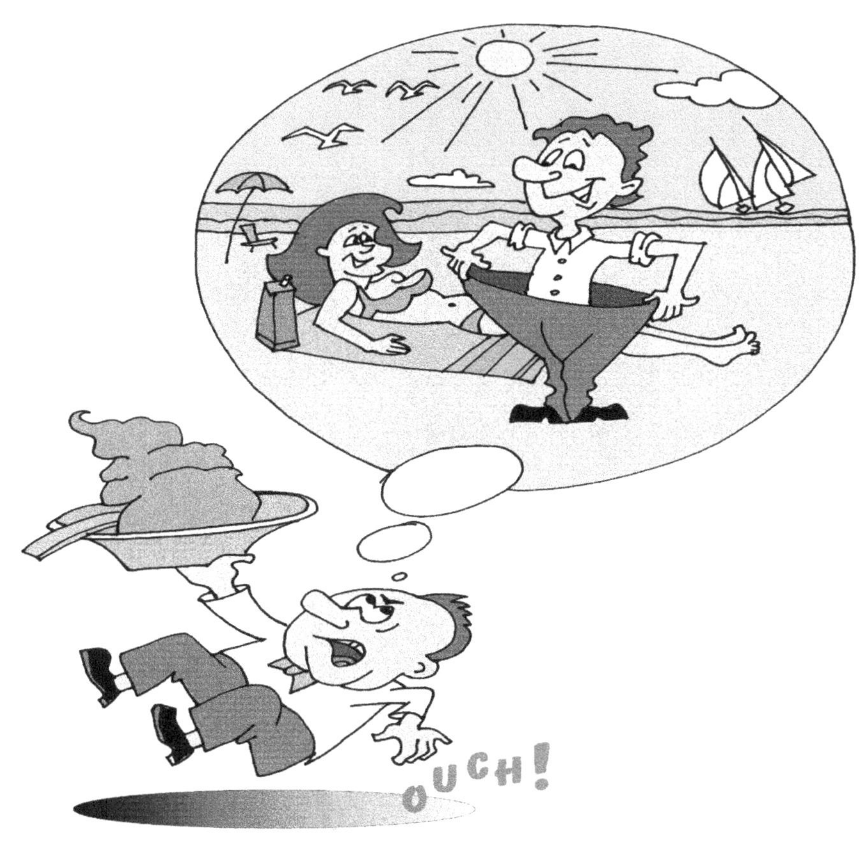

Chapter 6

Don't Eat Wrong—Long

"EYEBALLS OPEN, SLIMEBALL?"

You have your menu and your substitutes of low carborie FAVES. You also know that SLIP HAPPENS—you won't be perfect.

"When you fall off your horse, COWBOY, don't waste time getting back in control of your waist!"

Sergeant Otto has made you a list of new habits to reduce the time until you reach your goal. The more of these you choose, the sooner your scale gives good news.

A. Most parties involve alcohol. The problem with beer is that it sucks when it's warm. You can't nurse a warm beer. But you can *sip one glass of red wine all night*. Forget the "I'll have another cold one." Find a red wine that you like and add it to your list of FAVES.

"Wine tastes better with age. The older you get, the more you'll like it."

One glass (well, maybe two)—all night. Don't turn your parties into your "unhappy hour" and ruin your diet plan, Noah.

"No need to get shit-faced, PRINCESS. After you hit your goal and feel great, that's when you celebrate!"

B. *Raise your shelf esteem!* Look in the refrigerator and pantry. You wouldn't be reading this if you could easily resist the temptations of the variety of food. Either purge the junk or make a corner of the pantry and fridge that is just for your low carborie FAVES. Your food doesn't need to be scattered everywhere. Your shelf, your FAVES.

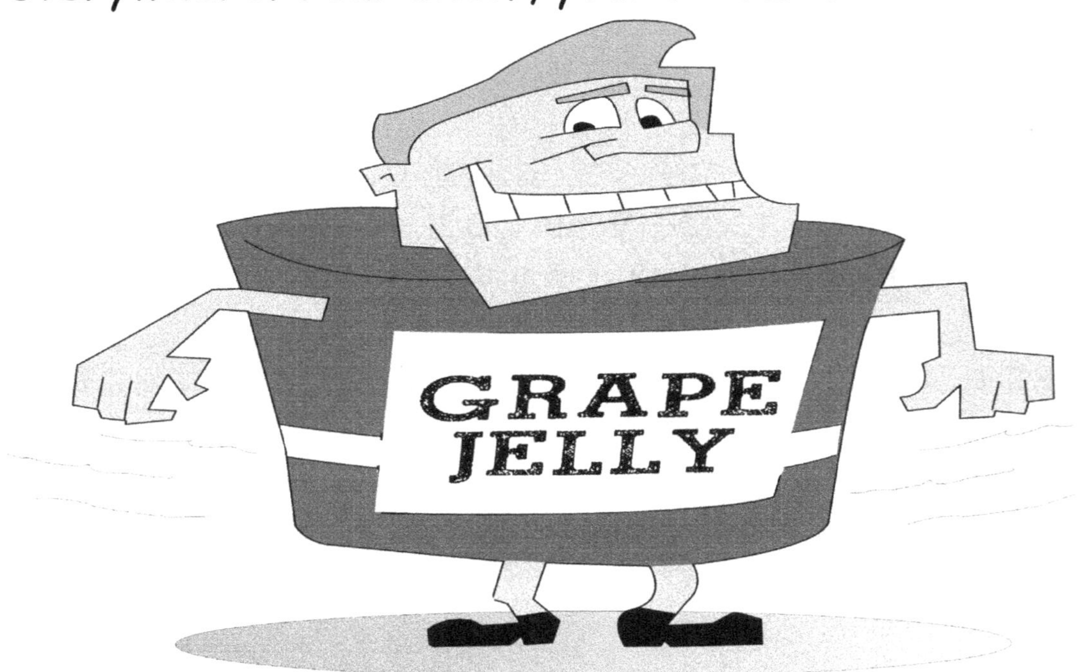

"Your shelf esteem is on the way up, JELLYBELLY!"

C. *Competition* will keep you focused on your mantra. Get a partner—wife, BFF, co-worker, neighbor. Share the experience. You will learn new habits together. But no partner? Screw it—just do it yourself.

"DELAYING IS UNACCEPTABLE!"

D. *No hoovering*—don't inhale your food. Whoa! Take it easy, slow down. You are eating less, enjoy it more.

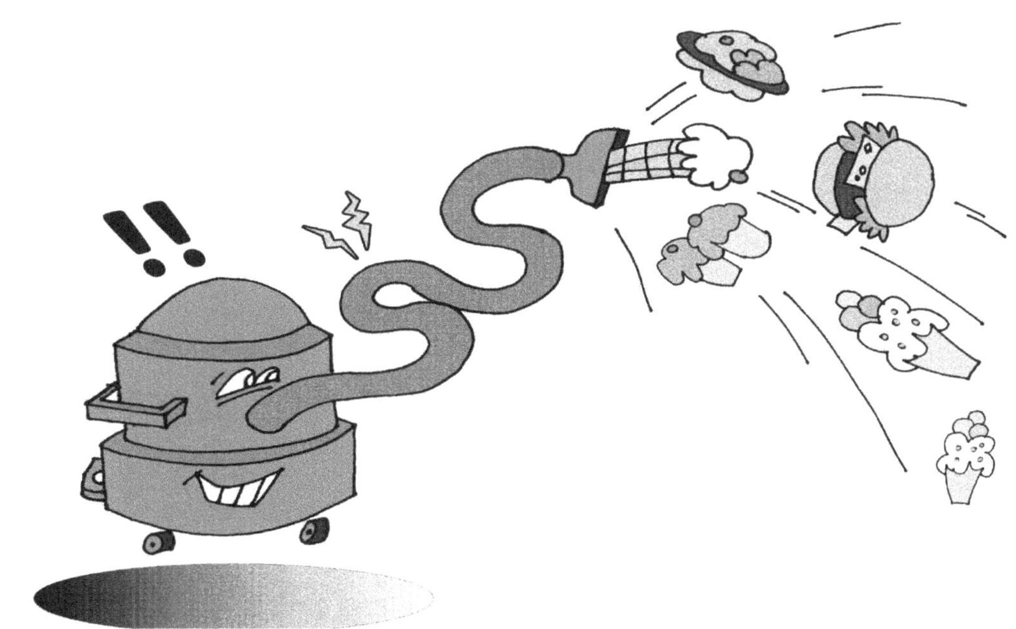

"Hoovering your snacks means bigger slacks!"

E. *Change your home page to www.menshealth.com*. There are always articles about health, weight, lifestyles. You may find new ideas that work for you. Use your computer to help get closer to your goals.

F. *No more chip tease!* If chips are on your list of FAVES then buy the small bag—you can eat the whole thing—you do not have to choose when to stop eating. You have a choice—eat the small bag or eat the big, old bag.

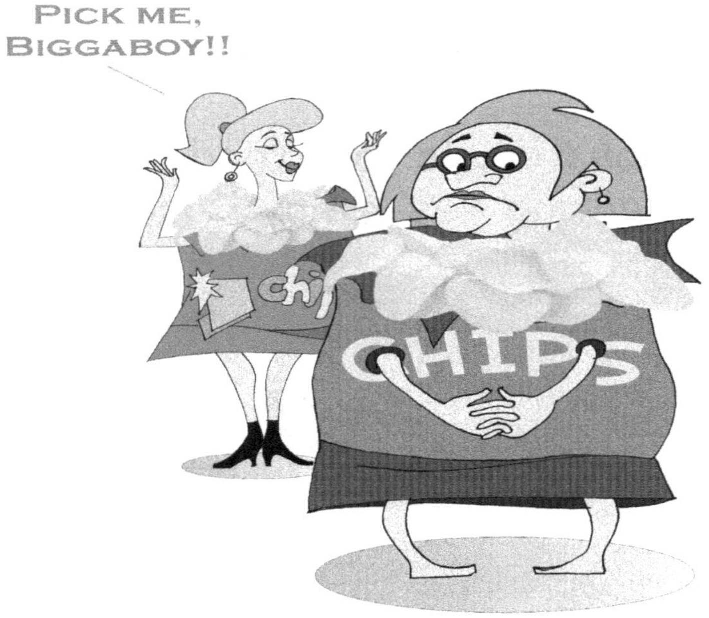

"I SAID EAT THE SMALL BAG, BUTTHEAD!"

"Always buy the small size of your snack FAVES!"

G. Put a *"HungerSpanker"* on your FAVES list. Own a Keurig? Try coffee and a dab of flavored creamer. To me, Keurig is, indeed, a special K!

"Find that low carborie 'HungerSpanker' that gets rid of the munchies for you, CANDYASS!"

H. As you are getting more serious about losing that gut, *build a 'Step-n-Work'.™*

"DON'T SIT, GET FIT!"

You can purchase a mini-stepper for $80 from a sporting goods retailer or Sears. Then find a box or shelf to raise your computer to a comfortable working and standing height.

Every minute that you're working at the computer you can be slowly walking. After a short time you will easily Step-n-Work for five to six hours a day—no problem. Give yourself a grade of "A-freakin'-plus" for your commitment to Sergeant Otto! See more details at the Step-n-Work tab at www.sgtotto.com.

If you Step-n-Work at your office, you will be a role model for all the fatsos at your workplace. And for once your boss-hole will be proud of your efforts!

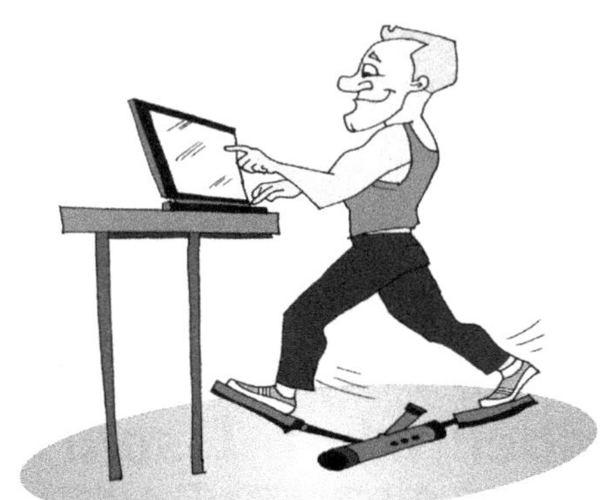

"JUST STEP-N-WORK, YA JERK!"

I. Need an aid to help *relearn portion control?* If cereal is on your list of FAVES, let the package determine your portion size.

"Buy the individual serving size cereal box not the standard larger size, LUNCHBOX."

If you finish off one small box of cereal every day for a year or two, who knows, you just might become a **famous cereal killer!**

J. Still looking for *low carborie snacks and foods* that you love? Consider these three...

Can't Beat My Meat!

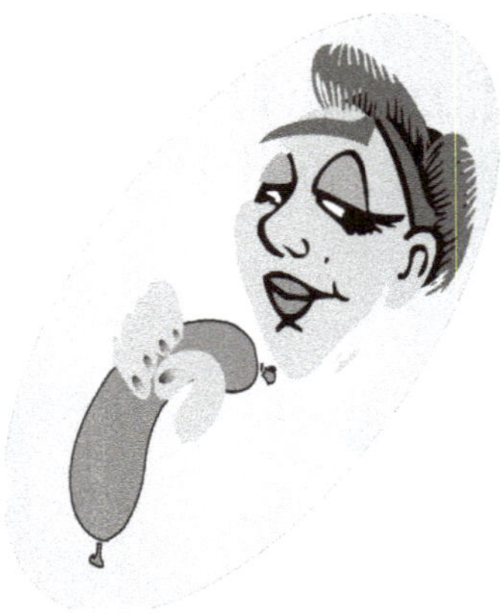

Like meat?
Wanna tasty treat?
Try a slice or two of salami,
Or maybe you prefer pastrami.
Don't like either?
Then go suck on a wiener!
Minimal carbs, minimal cals,
Make these three your secret pals.
Just remember what I said,
Thou shalt eat NO FREAKIN' BREAD!

K. As your weight comes down, others will start making positive comments about the *"NewYou"*.

"No more MASTER-DATING, doing things alone. It is time to get out and be more social."

L. *Be loyal to foods that spoil!* Anything on your FAVES list that can spoil? Apples, bananas, cauliflower, grapes, carrots, cucumbers—there is a long list of foods. If it can spoil, it is good for you.

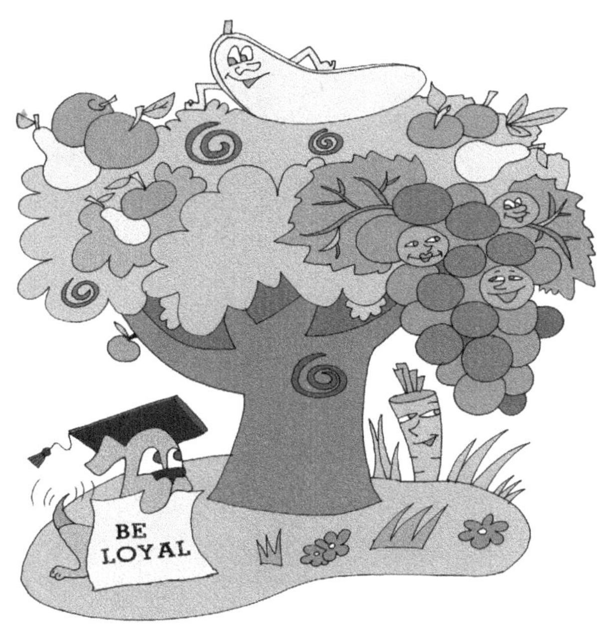

"Got 'spoilers' on your FAVES list?"

"IF NOT, ADD THE 'SPOILERS' YOU LOVE TO YOUR LOW CARBORIE MENU, BUTTMUNCHER!"

M. *What about desserts?* You can still buy those things. The trick is to then give it to friends, family, co-workers. You will get the hugs and feel the love. Make their day while you walk away! Let **them** scarf it down!

"Are you nucking futs to buy donuts, pizza, cake, pie, ice cream?"

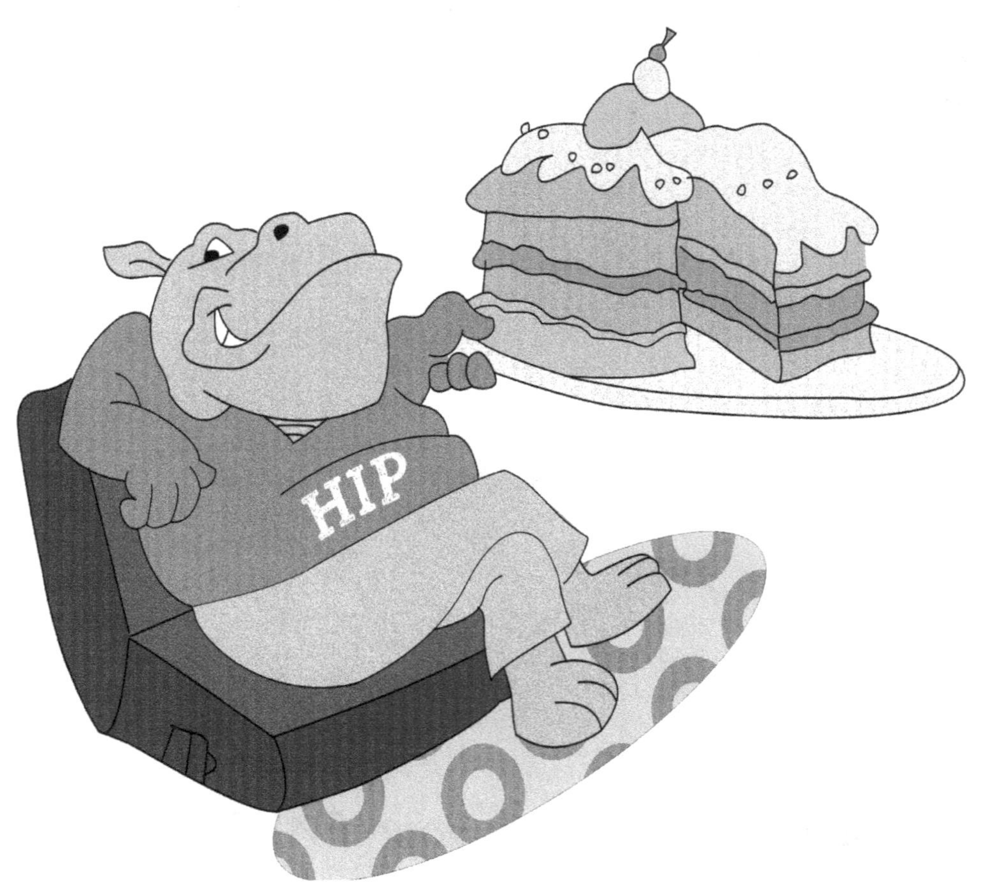

"No, the secret is to buy—NOT EAT, HIPPO!"

"Just bring it...!"

N. If today you fought the temptations, did not commit *"FoodSin,"* and were faithful to your FAVES *"FoodBible,"* then *you deserve a tasty dessert* that won't eff up your plan. Try Instant Jell-O Pudding, sugar and fat free. Add Cool Whip Lite topping—total of nine carbs and ninety calories.

"Ya' startin' to look 'be-u-ti-mus,' SWEETPEA!"

And then each time you lose ten,
Go ahead—dive in.
Hit that springboard.
You deserve a decadent reward.

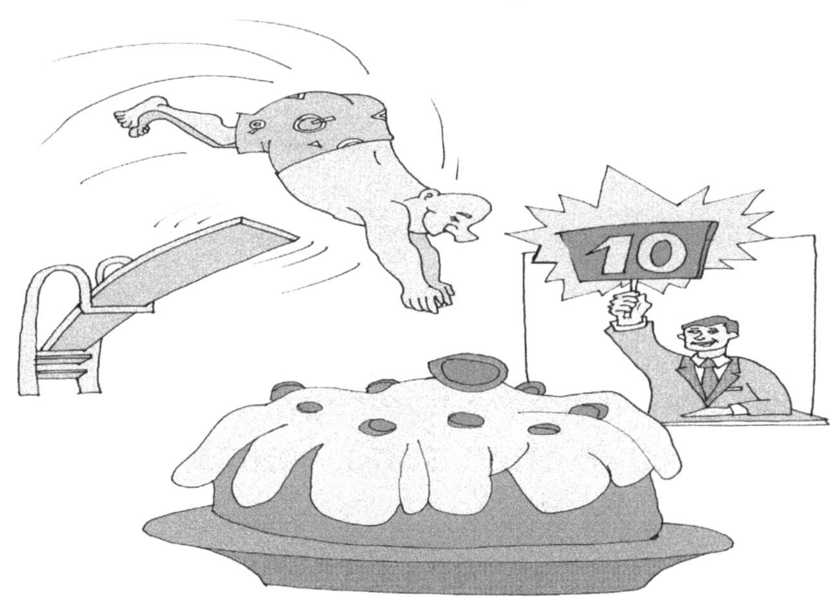

"You don't need Sergeant Otto telling you what to do.
Next meal, get back to your freakin' menu!"

O. If you find yourself *falling behind* your schedule of weight loss, look for other FAVES.

DON'T BITE THE WHITE

STOP the sugar, daddy!
RESIST flour power!
HALT the salt!
NO-NO on the potato!

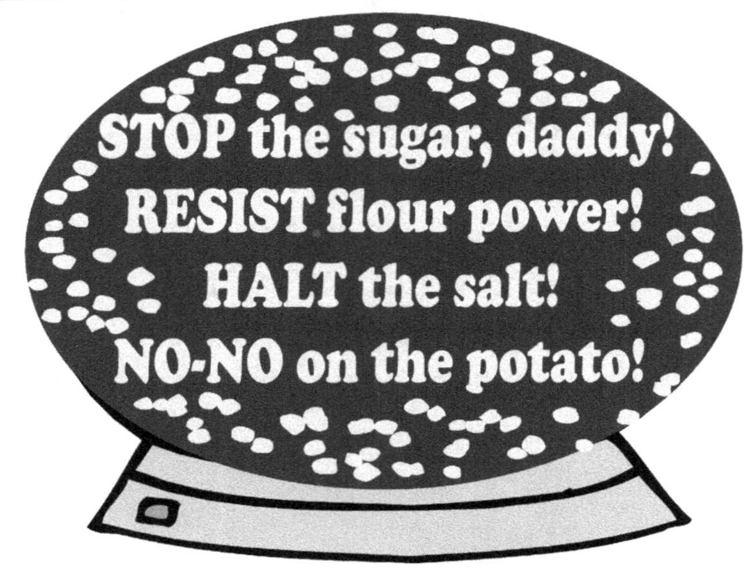

THESE RULES ARE HELPFUL TOOLS

P. *Drink more water.* Okay, that's easier said than done. If you try Kraft MiO, Propel Zero or other water additives,you may have found another *"HungerSpanker."* These taste great and are less expensive than soda. Remember Mikey? "Try it, you'll like it."

Q. *Get Rigid!* Find your low carborie lunch FAVE and remember—variety is the **vice**.... You know the drill by now. Monday through Friday I ate the same low carborie lunch every day for seven months. You can do the same with your FAVES until you reach your goal.

R. Because of the reduced variety and repetitive eating of the same foods week after week, *carborie counting is easy*. Record the carbories of all items in your weekly menu by installing the My Fitness Pal app. Track your calories and carbs per meal, per day, and per week. This will get you focused **and** keep you focused. If you do nothing else suggested in this book, **you must do this!**

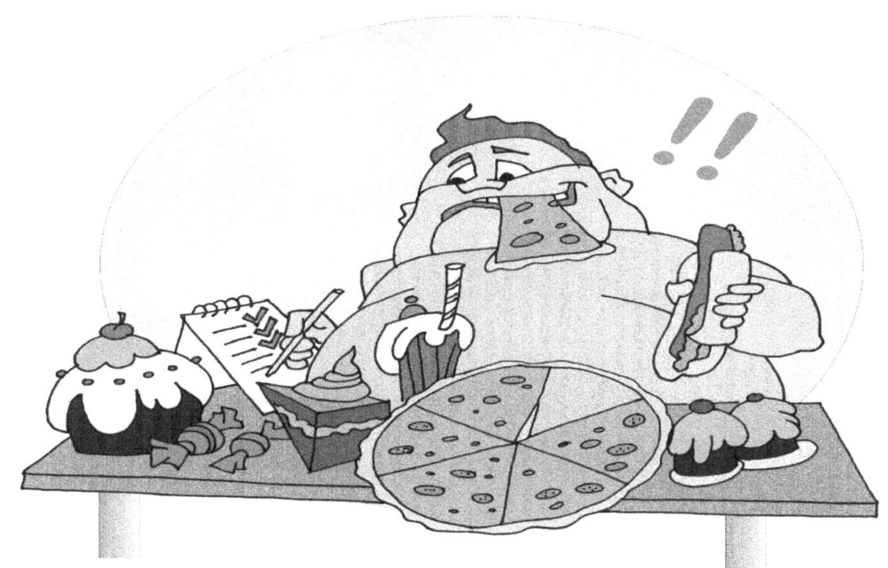

"START RECORDING EVERYTHING YOU EAT."

"You can record the carbories of a meal in less than 30 seconds while stuffing your kisser, FATBUTT!"

"When you stick it in your mouth, stick it in your phone, GOOBER."

S. *Observe but don't swerve.* If you find yourself in a crowd with none of your FAVES in sight, then look at the plates of the skinny people—just eat what they eat.

***"Look at the plates of the 'phatsos'—
DON'T EAT THAT CRAP!"***

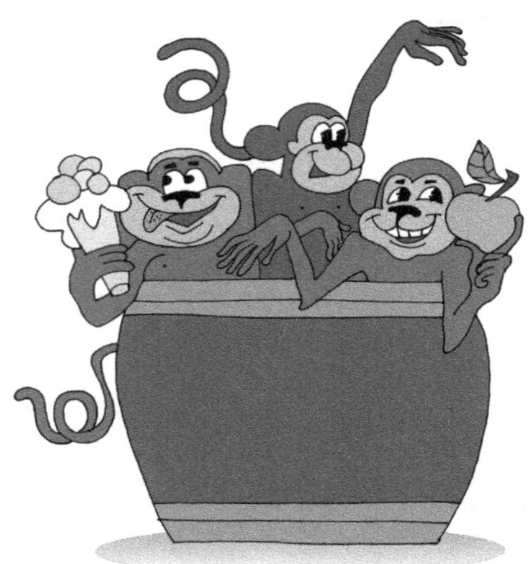

"Monkey See, Monkey Do!"

T. *Start reading the nutrition labels* on food packages when you are at the grocery store. Check out the carbories per serving on the packages. The print is very small. Warning! Some things you do may cause blindness.

***"Remember what yer momma told you causes blindness,
JAGOFF?"***

Well, reading the small print of nutrition labels was **NOT** one of them!

"If you get behind on your schedule of weight loss, pay more attention to the labels, change your weekly menu to other FAVES, and reduce your carbories."

U. If you are unable to avoid fast food joints, just order from their healthy menu items. *McD, BK, Taco Bell have reduced carborie foods.* Look on-line, find the best for you.

"Plan ahead. It wasn't raining when.... Oh, you've heard it before. Go Noah!"

V. *Proudly display your weekly menu.* Good spots to hang it include your refrigerator door, pantry door, bathroom mirror, and near your scale.

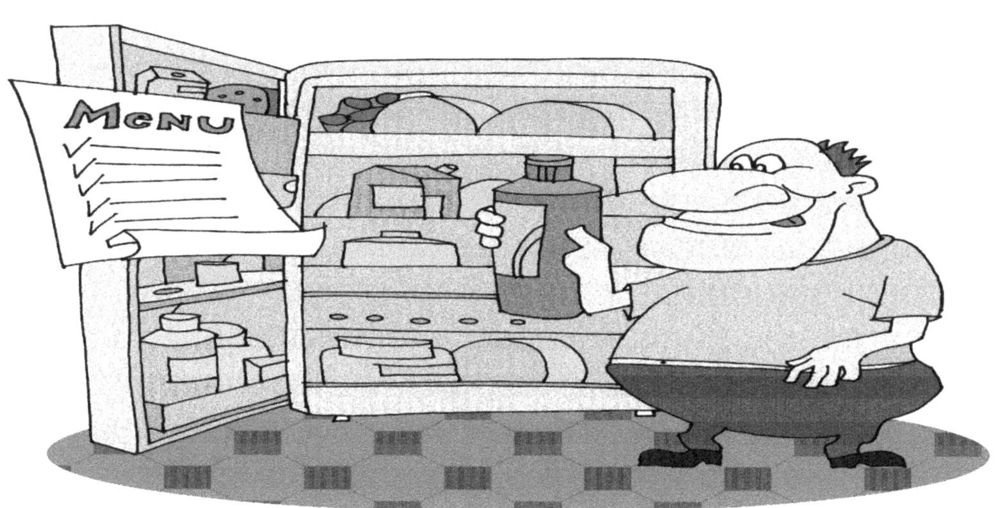

"JUST FOLLOW YOUR DAILY MENU, BLUBBER BOY!"

Chapter 7

What the Pho?

"You need 'HabitBusters' to change years of racking up the pounds!"

If you do a little soul-searching, you **know** the benefits of being trim far exceed the temporary comforts associated with poor eating choices.

But the large quantity of information, changes, and choices presented earlier could cause you to postpone or never start this program. The next five lines condense the message in this manual with the hope that this simplified explanation will stimulate your desire to **get started now!**

1. Set a realistic goal and ending date—**mantra**.

2. Create a list of FAVES—**love them or leave them**.

3. Eliminate high carb-calorie (carborie) foods from your FAVES list. Remember—**variety is the VICE of life**.

4. Make a **weekly lower carborie FAVES MENU** of meals and snacks then start recording everything you eat.

5. **Repeat your weekly menu** until you reach your goal!

"Adopt the new habits from chapter six, then you'll start getting the chicks!"

"FINISH THE NEXT TWO CHAPTERS AND THEN READ THIS BOOK AGAIN, FLABSTER."

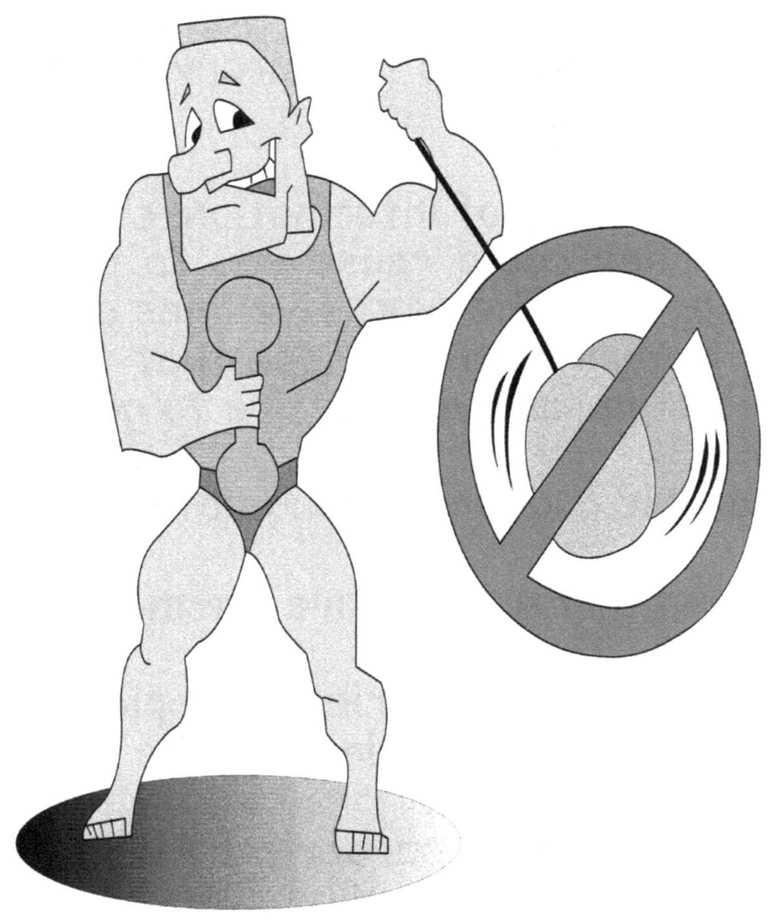

"What the Pho? No more Yo-Yo!"

Chapter 8

Drill Baby Drill!

"Ok TUBS, you're headed in the right direction, making good choices, eating only low carborie foods you love. Just keep 'milking that cow'."

"Flush those bad habits, GRUNT—keep it up."

SLIP HAPPENS but you always get back in control. You are looking better. Time to buy a new shirt.

"HAL-LA-FREAKIN'-LOO-YA!"

"A new smaller size shirt—your first badge of achievement!"

"Feelin' good, CASANOVA? Hell yeaa-AH!"

As you gradually 'shrink' you will also start using new holes in your belt. But whoa, hold on—at some point no more belt holes! What now—time for a new belt?

"SCREW YOU, MAN!"

"ABSOLUTELY DO NOT BUY A NEW BELT!"

"Get your drill and make your OWN holes in that old belt and then wear it every day!"

Every morning you'll get a reminder of your success and hard work. Your belt is getting a longer tail!

"That belt tail is another badge of achievement, TWINKIE!"

"Take a photo, send it to me, Sergeant Otto. I'm waiting."

"Cheech and Chong were wrong. You DO need 'stinkin' baudges' mawn!"

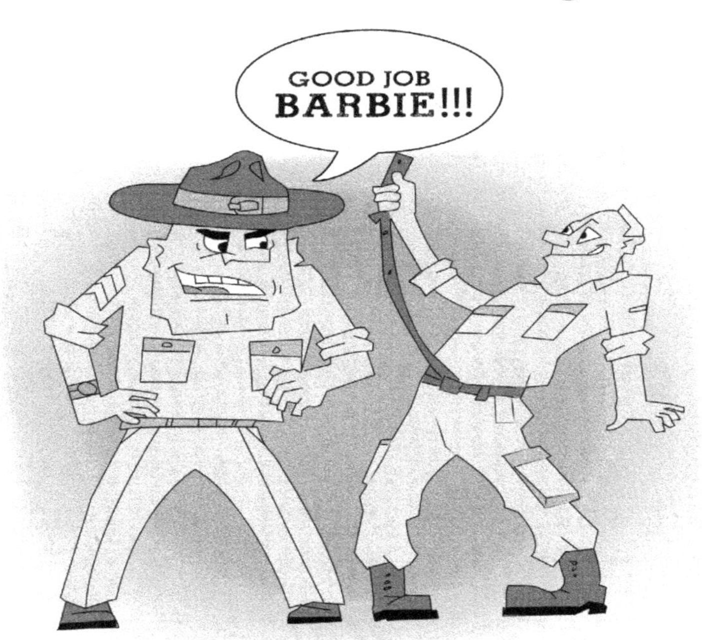

"Get svelte, watch that blubber melt, then drill that belt."

"JUST DRILL BABY DRILL!"

Chapter 9

Bite Me, Less.

"Read on, PLUMPKIN."

So what is the payoff after adopting Sergeant Otto's "less variety" philosophy?

1. Less variety means *more cash*. Did you know that fatsos earn less? Fatsos make less "dough". If you want your income to go up, get your weight down.

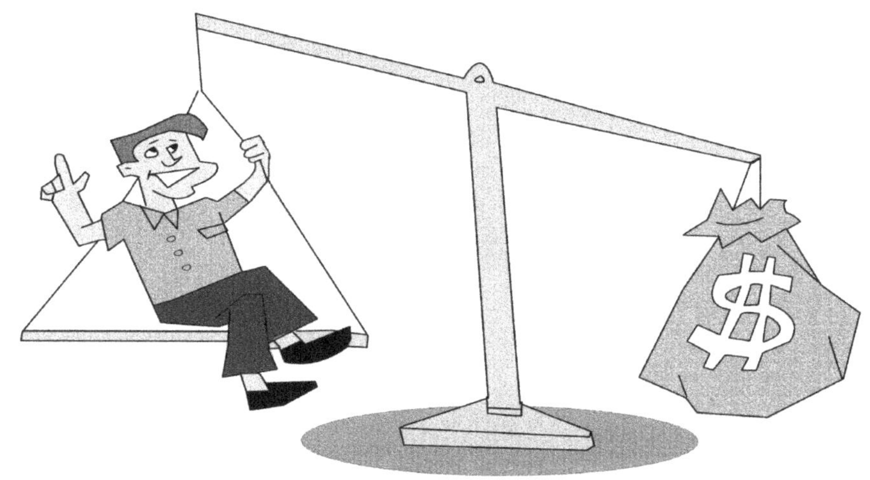

"Get more cash with less gut! Don't believe?"

"Google it, MR. BAITER!"

2. *Getting laid* is invigorating. The more you hide the salami, the happier you are. The happier you are, the healthier you become. The healthier you become, the more you hide the salami.

"If you want some quickies, reduce those carbories!"

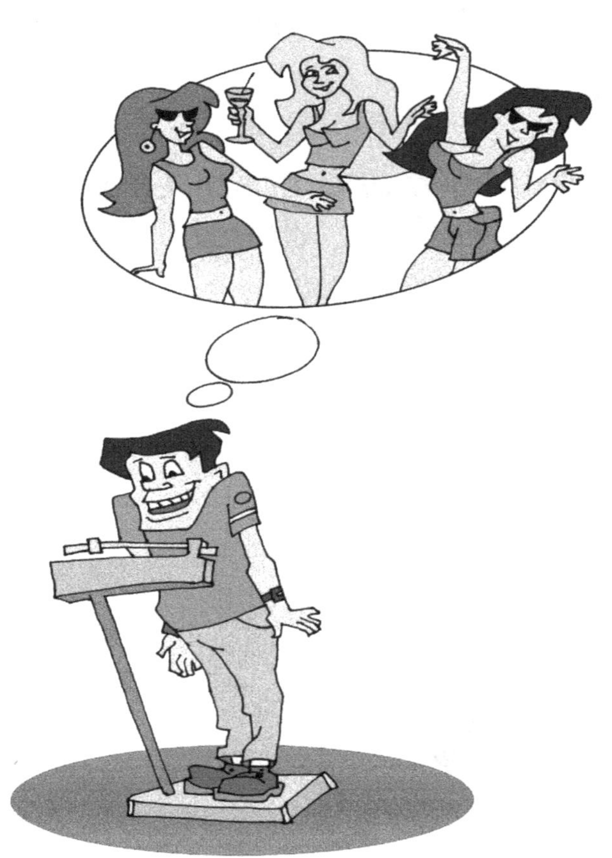

"Get more nookie with less gut! Don't believe?"

"Google that, BLUBBA!"

3. Less variety means more years. No secret here. If you control your weight, you will *live longer*.

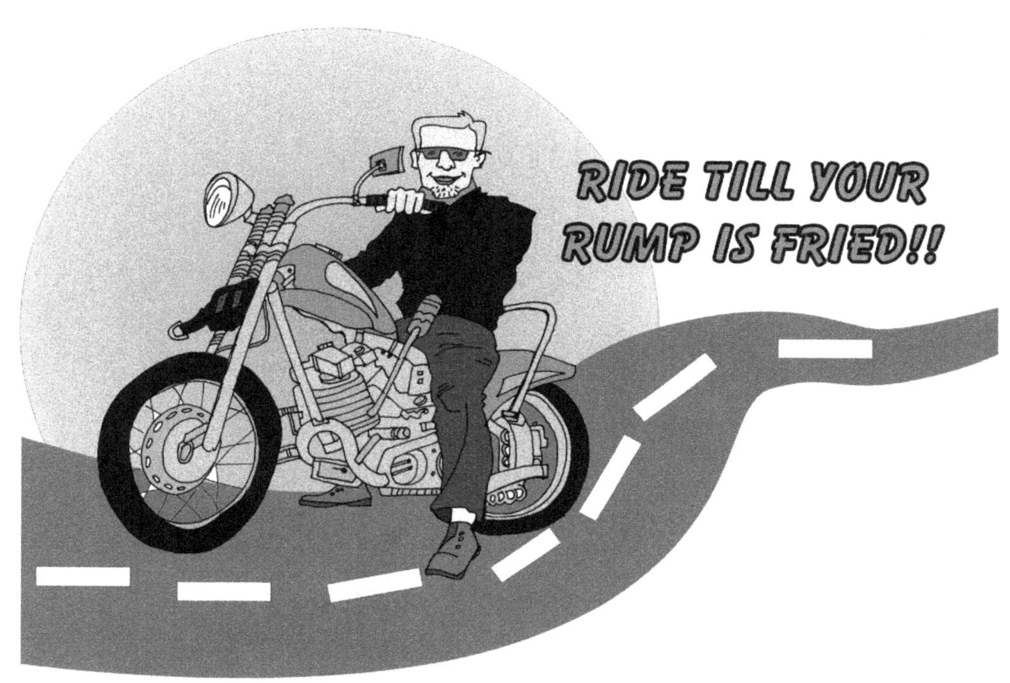

"Get older with less gut! Don't believe?"

"Google it, GENIUS!"

Not a bad list above. Lose weight and get more money, get more sex, and get more years!

And there is ONE MORE WELL DOCUMENTED AND UNEXPECTED MEDICAL BENEFIT of significant weight loss...

4. Get a drastic *improvement in eyesight!* As your gut slowly disappears and you are getting close to your goal, call an optometrist. When the receptionist answers, speak very loudly into the phone...

I CAN SEE MY WEENER!
!!!
I BEG YOUR PARDON, PERV!
RECEPTIONIST

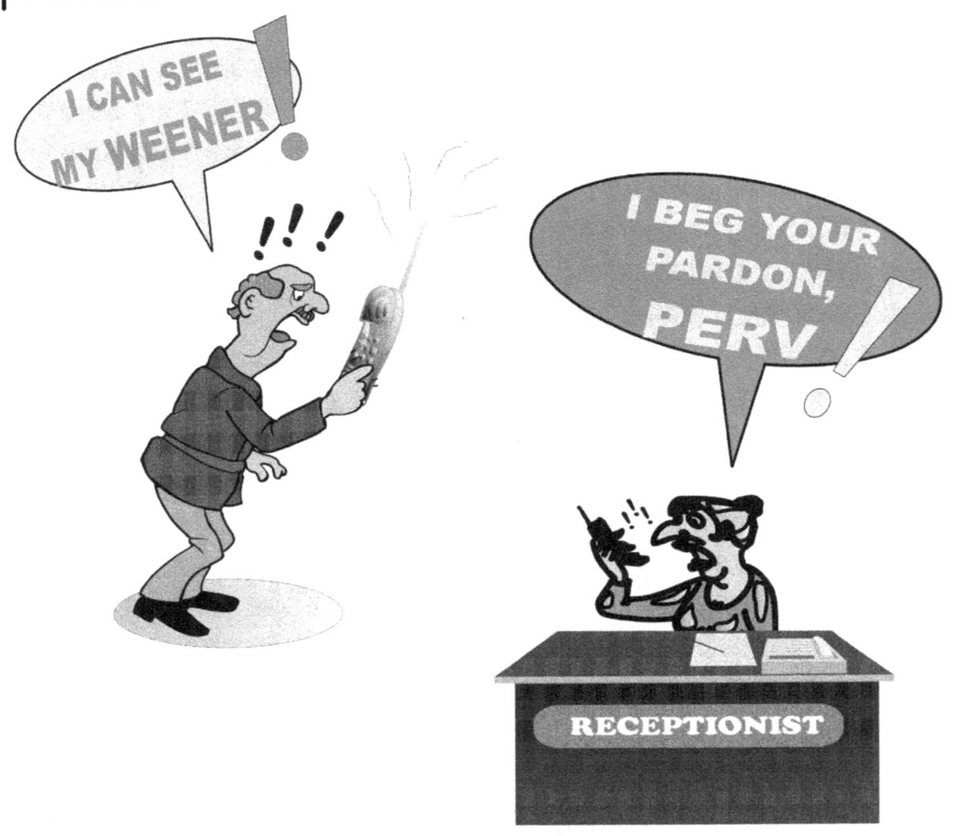

"When WAS the last time you saw your weener, BLIMPO?"

You knew it was there—you could touch it, but with that gut you just couldn't see it! Get better vision with less gut!

"And don't bother to Google it, ya' IGNOR-ANUS!"

My FAVES Weekly Menu

NOW GO FILL IN YOURS

	M	T	W	TH	F	S	S
Breakfast	1 Egg Banana	same	same	same	same	Omelet	Omelet
Lunch	Coke Zero Beef Jerky	same	same	same	same	pick below	pick below
Dinner	Chef Salad	Grilled Tuna	2 Burger Patties	Chicken Salad	Grilled Chicken	Salmon Steak	Beef Filet
Dessert	Pudding Cool Whip	none	same	none	same	same	none

Snack and meal compliments to plug into weekly menu:

grapes cauliflower baby carrots watermelon
cheese nuts Jell-O red wine deviled eggs wings
pepperoni hot dog sausage salami

Record all your carbories to track your progress. You determine food portion size depending on your daily carborie goals and if you are ahead or behind schedule—your mantra.

"IT'S ONLY TEMPORARY, LOVERBOY!"

"WHAT'S YOUR MANTRA, DINGLEBERRY?"

"REMEMBER VARIETY IS THE VICE OF LIFE, PECKERHEAD!"

"LOVE IT OR LEAVE IT, LAMEASS!"

"NOW DO IT, LOSE THAT WEIGHT—FOR YOUR COUNTRY, FOR SERGEANT OTTO, AND FOR YER MOMMA!"

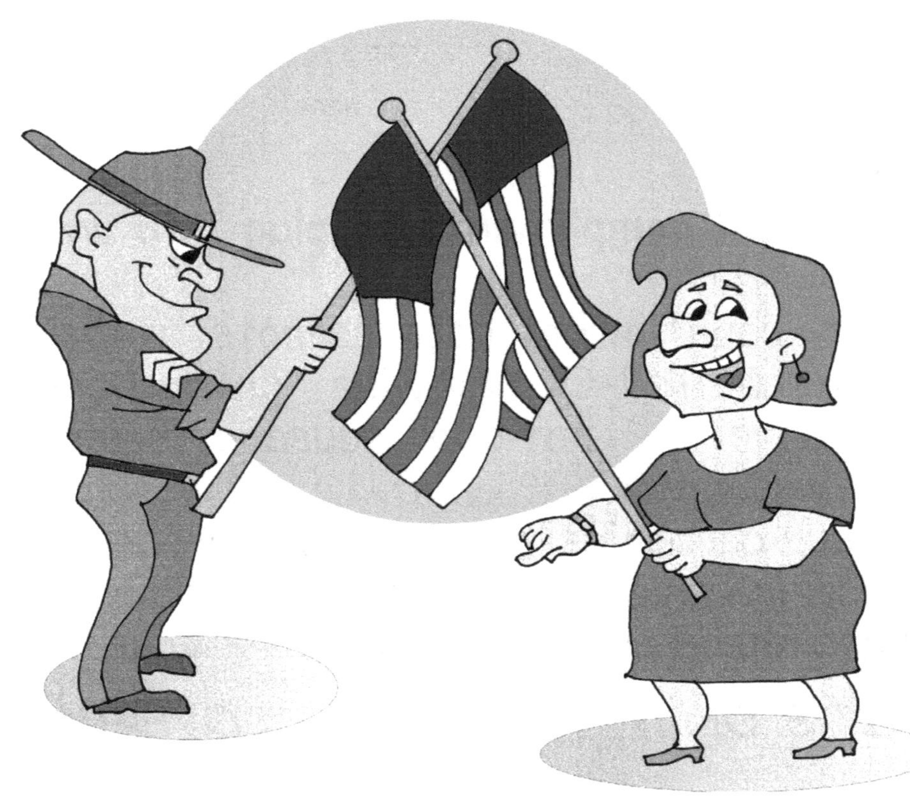

As Arnold Schwarzenegger says, **"The best activities in life are pumping and humping."** You will be doing a lot more of both as you reach your goal!

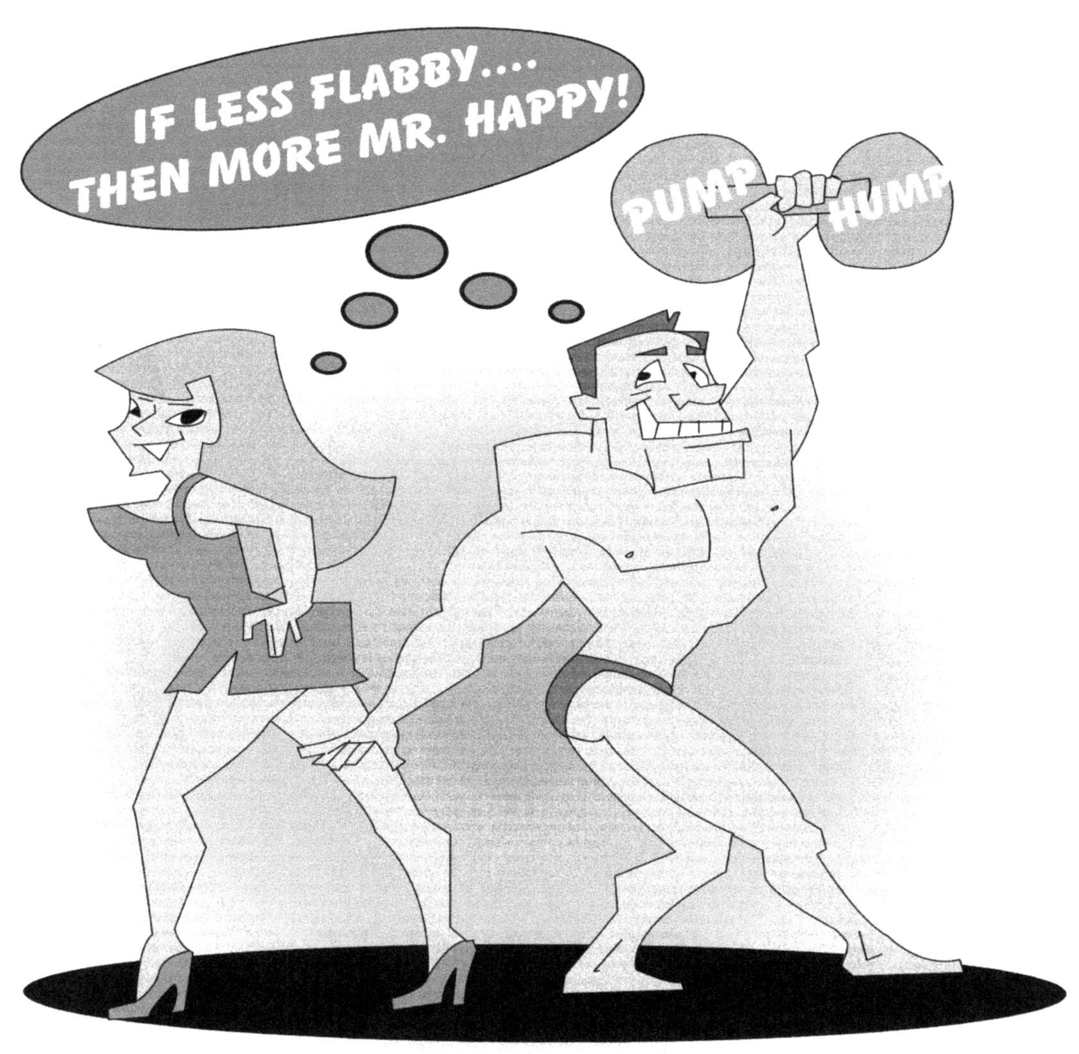

"IT'S TIME!"

"ALL THOSE IN FAVOR OF SERGEANT OTTO PLEASE RISE!"

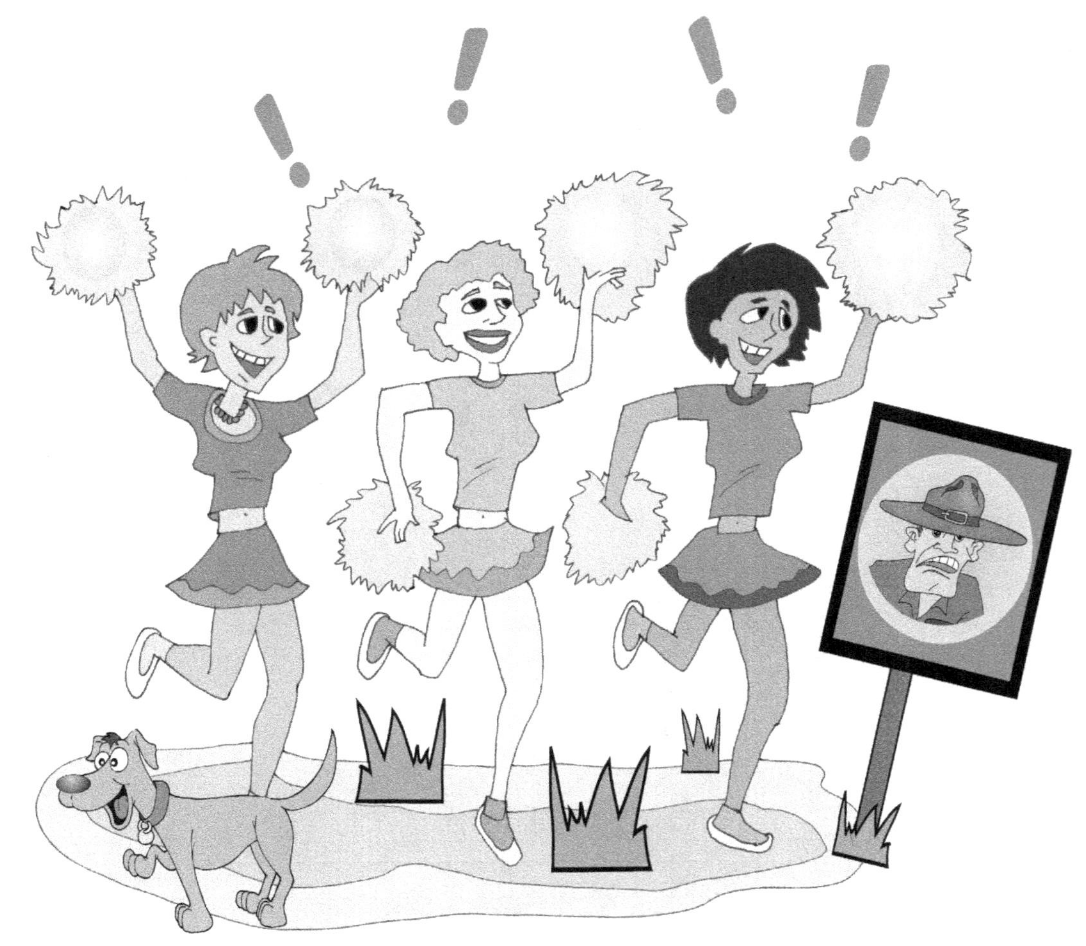

"NOW GET BUSY, YOU AIN'T GETTIN' ANY YOUNGER, YANKER!"

"DO THE WRITING ASSIGNMENTS!"

"READ THIS MANUAL AGAIN!"

"START WORK ON THE NEW HABITS, THE MORE OF THOSE YOU CHOOSE, THE FASTER YOU WILL LOSE!"

"If you are zealous, others will be jealous!"

"See ya' at www.sgtotto.com."

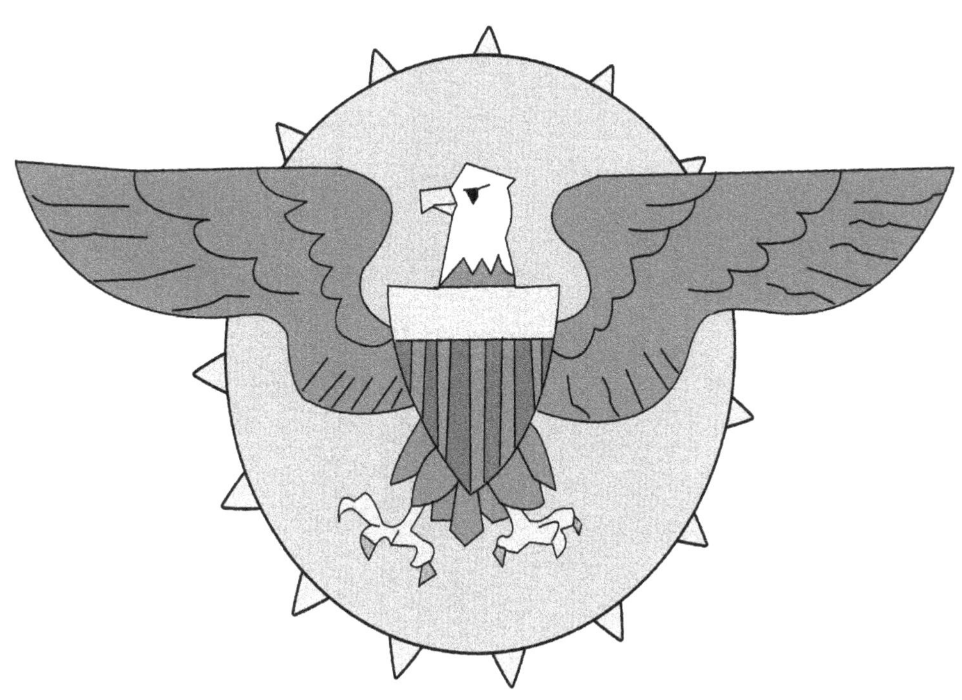

"AMEN, MY CHUNKY BROTHER, AMEN!"

www.sgtotto.com

You will find...

1. Sgt. Otto Man Diet (R-rated). Weight loss guide with aggressive military language and adult cartoons. Digital and paperback copies available.

2. Sgt. Otto Diet Advice (PG-rated). Same weight loss message as Man Diet, but aggressive language and adult cartoons removed. Your grandma could read it! Digital and paperback formats available.

3. Sgt. Otto logo items to be used as reminders to keep you focused.

4. Getting Started—guided planning, follow-through, goal attainment.

5. About the Author.

6. The Healthy University—free Permanently Healthy Diploma (PHD).

7. Link to Facebook, Twitter, and blog.

8. Details of Step-n-Work.

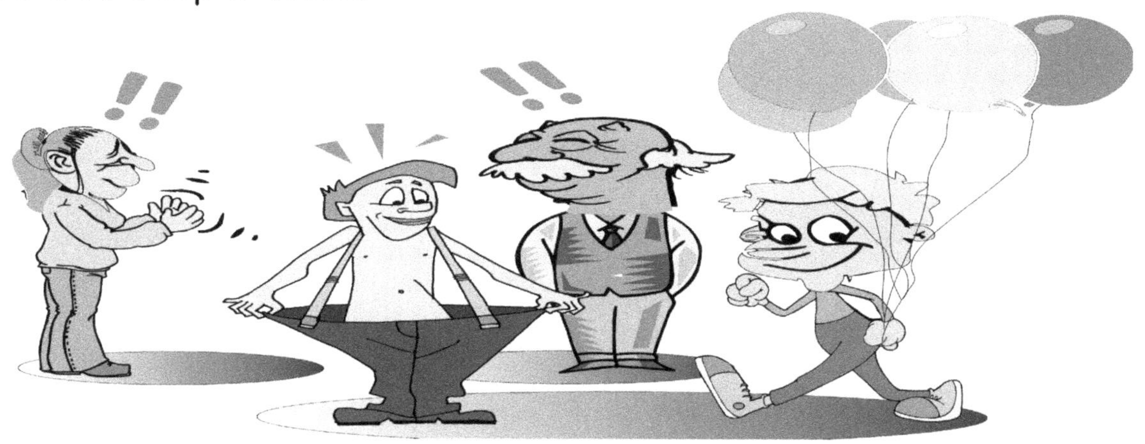

"After you have made good food choices,
Your friends will cheer and make loud noises!"

Current and Upcoming Cartoon Publications

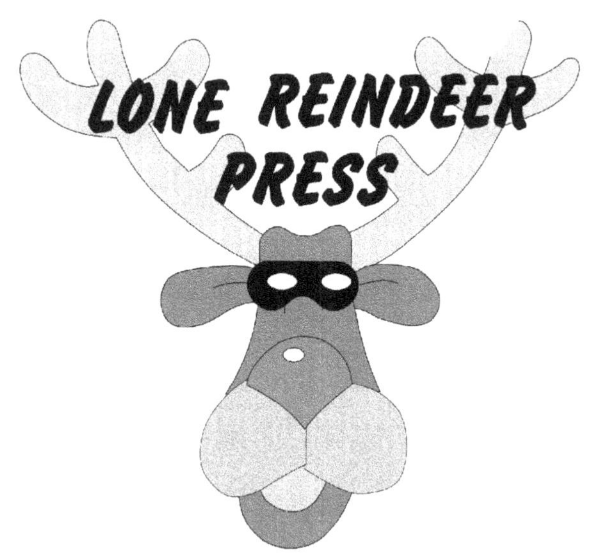

Sergeant Otto Man Diet
Diet guidelines, adult cartoons, aggressive language,
R-rated (2014)

Sergeant Otto Diet Advice
Same diet message, adult cartoons and language removed,
PG-rated (2014)

Sergeant Otto Woman Diet
(Winter 2015)

Sergeant Otto HOOAH Cookbook
(Spring 2016)

www.ingramcontent.com/pod-product-compliance
Lightning Source LLC
Chambersburg PA
CBHW081650270326
41933CB00018B/3412
* 9 7 8 0 9 8 9 7 6 1 9 3 2 *